GV
697
A1
D29
1993

Darden, Bob
December champions

DATE DUE			

DECEMBER CHAMPIONS

BY BOB DARDEN AND W. R. SPENCE, M.D.

WRS
PUBLISHING

A Division of WRS Group, Inc.
Waco, Texas

First published in the United States of America in 1993 by WRS Publishing,
A Division of WRS Group, Inc., 701 N. New Road, Waco, Texas 76710.
Book design by Kenneth Turbeville
Jacket design by Talmage Minter and Joe James

10 9 8 7 6 5 4 3 2 1

Library of Congress Cataloging-in-Publication Data

Darden, Bob, 1954–
    December champions / by Bob Darden and W.R. Spence.
        p.   cm.
    ISBN 1-56796-008-1 : $19.95
    1. Aged athletes—United States—Biography. 2. Sports for the aged—
United States. I. Spence, Wayman. II. Title.
GV697.A1D29 1993
796'.092'2—dc20
    [B]
                                                                    93–8960
                                                                        CIP

Table of Contents

Dedication

December Champions is dedicated to my grandmother,
Mrs. Allie Owens of Woodville, Texas — Bob Darden

Special Thanks

Bob Darden would like to thank Ann Page of WRS
Publishing for her invaluable assistance in locating and
contacting the 25 splendid athletes and human beings
who comprise *December Champions.*

Foreword

They personify my philosophy of life: Anything is possible! Make it happen!

The December champions portrayed in this book should serve as inspiration to anyone—at any age. They are to be commended for not giving up and for not giving in. Old age has not slowed them down, it has just given them more time to accomplish their goals. It has not left them sitting on a front porch somewhere enjoying their rocking chairs. It has sent them to the softball fields or the polo grounds or the mountains... or anywhere they choose to spend their time enjoying life to the fullest.

Pride and discipline are required if we are to be successful in business or in our personal lives. The people featured in this book exemplify the remarkable achievements made possible by maintaining pride and discipline.

Congratulations to every December champion around the world! I hope that everyone who reads this book will be inspired by the knowledge that nothing is impossible. It is never too late to make changes in your own life. Learn from the examples in this book; set your own goals, and work to accomplish them—just as these December champions have done.

BY JACK LALANNE

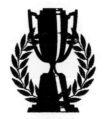

Introduction

December Champions isn't about old people. It is about people who have radically, dynamically taken control of their lives. It is—with only a couple of exceptions—about men and women who, at some point in their lives, decided to just do it. If there is a theme running through the 25 interviews that comprise *December Champions*, it is exactly that: *Go ahead and do it!*

Do what? Barefoot water-ski, compete in the Ironman Triathlon, run marathons, parachute out of airplanes, play polo, swim marathons, run sprints, race automobiles, windsurf, ride in bicycle marathons, rope calves, or race around barrels, play softball, climb mountains, dance, coach cross-country, play tennis, play racquetball. *Go ahead and do it!*

People's lives don't end at age 65. Or 55, for that matter. That's only the first lap. After all, the Census Bureau reports that the United States now has 106,000 people over 100. By the year 2000, more than 13 percent of the population will be over 65, according to the U.S. Public Health Service.

If "Go ahead and do it!" is the theme, this is the chorus:

You *can* do it.

And you can do it *now*.

It is never too late to start.

Nobody profiled in *December Champions* ran a marathon the first day. Some had trouble walking around the block the first day. Both the marathon and the block began the same way: With a single step. But before the Step there was the Thought: *Go ahead and do it!*

No one disputes that taking that first step is difficult. But as Richard Bohannon, an 84-year-old physician in Dallas who has walked or jogged for about two miles, six mornings a week for 30 years, told *The New York Times:* "I just always think about my motto. The devil can't hit a moving target."

Without exception, these 25 athletes look, act, think, and feel younger than their rocking chair–bound peers. What many have instinctively known for years is now being proven in the halls of science and research. These 25—and the thousands like them—don't just look and think younger, they *are* younger. Not only are they living longer, they're living *better*. They've learned what science has now proven: Old age is *not* a disease. Individual organs, individual systems may have diseases, but old age is not a disease. Proper care of organs and systems will prevent most of those diseases. Or, as Dr. John Rowe, president of Mount Sinai Medical Center in New York, puts it: decline and disease are simply *not* the same thing.

Some things—inherited defects or predispositions, accidents, incurable diseases—cannot be avoided.

Virtually everything else can.

In fact, Dr. Mark H. Beers, assistant professor of medicine in geriatrics and gerontology at UCLA Medical Center and co-author of *Aging in Good Health*, says that if your doctor attributes something to aging, be wary.

"Very few symptomatic complaints are attributable to aging alone," Dr. Beers said. "Consider seeing another doctor, preferably a geriatric specialist."

California physician Walter Bortz II, former president of the American Geriatrics Society, echoes the same sentiment: "Most of what we think about aging is wrong. Most declines people consider inevitable are actually a result of disuse. Too often aging is a self-fulfilling prophecy... Aging happens, but it happens at a much more rapid rate if you're unfit."

In the *Age Wave* by Dr. Ken Dychtwald and Joe Flower, there is a story about an 82-year-old man who visits a doctor because of pain in his left knee:

"The doctor examines it and says, 'Well, what do you expect? After all, it's an 82-year-old knee.'

'Sure it is,' says the patient. 'But my right knee is also 82, and it's not bothering me a bit.'"

According to Dr. Dychtwald, 80 percent of the health problems of older people are now thought to be preventable or postponable. "What many of us call aging is a lifestyle issue."

The good news is that you don't *have* to run marathons to get into great shape. When Ginnie Wagner or Norton Davey say, "Go ahead and do it," they're talking about just a few simple changes that—if undertaken at *any* time in your life—

will, almost miraculously, alter your life forever. Those changes are: 1. Sustained physical activity. 2. Sustained mental activity. 3. A low-fat, healthy diet. 4. Companionship. 5. Luck.

Sustained physical activity

December Champions details the lives of 25 people, most of whom took up a rigorous physical activity in the later part of life that, in time, irrevocably changed their lives for the better.

* At 88, Lucille Thompson took up tae kwon do.

* At 70, fitness guru Jack LaLanne, shackled and handcuffed, towed 70 boats of friends and reporters in Long Beach Harbor.

* At 100, Claire Willi takes dance lessons.

* On her 88th birthday, Reva Coon took her first glider flight.

* At 73, Paul Reese ran across America in 124 days.

* At 90, Viola Krahn participates in competitive diving events.

* At 94, Frank Batchelder is still flying airplanes.

There are, perhaps, 100,000 equally fine examples.

Consider just one sport/activity that is finding renewed popularity among seniors: weight or strength training, also called bodybuilding or weight lifting. William Evans, chief of the human physiology lab at the Human Nutrition Research Center on Aging at Tufts University, believes that weight training is the single most critical factor in retarding the aging process. Evans cites recent studies that indicate that strength training can arrest—or even reverse—the aging process.

New studies from the National Institute on Aging have found that 90-year-olds can improve their leg strength by as much as 170 percent and their gait speed by 48 percent.

You don't have to pump iron, of course. The type of exercise simply doesn't matter, as long as you do *something.*

New Washington University School of Medicine studies indicate that people between the ages of 60 and 71 can improve their cardiovascular function by 20–25 percent in just one year through regular endurance exercise. This improvement is *comparable to that reported in much younger people.*

The landmark study on the subject, published in *The Journal of the American Medical Association* in 1989, reported that physical fitness—as measured with a treadmill test—was strongly related to the risk of death in seniors. More than 13,000 men and women were followed for an average of eight years by Steven N. Blair and his colleagues at the Cooper Institute for Aerobics Research in Dallas. According to Blair, the least fit groups had *substantially* higher death rates from all causes, especially from heart disease and cancer, than the most fit subjects.

"The greatest benefit comes to formerly sedentary people who start moving, even at a low intensity," Blair said.

Sustained mental activity

The second lifestyle change needed to ensure a long and vivacious life after the age of 60 involves the mental rather than the physical. Virginia Essex, initiative coordinator for the American Association of Retired Persons, believes that the two are inextricably related:

"When you give up on life, you bring on disabilities and poor health. Don't stop growing, learning, listening, asking questions, and sharing."

A study done at the National Institute on Aging found that the mind is more resilient than the body—it's the body that usually fails first. Recently published studies by Drs. K. Warner Schaie and Sherry Willis at Pennsylvania State University and Paul Baltes in Berlin indicate that not only can older people retain their memories, they can actually improve them. How? By using and exercising their powers of memorization and learning something new and challenging, like a musical instrument or a foreign language.

The mind is like any other muscle: use it or lose it.

Low-fat, healthy diet

All people, and particularly those over 50, need a diet high in nutrition, low-fat foods, beta-carotene, vitamins C and E, calcium, chromium, fiber, fluid, and other nutrients to help the body stay younger, healthier, and more flexible.

One of the intriguing trends which surfaced in *December Champions'* unscientific survey of 25 senior athletes is that most had either quit eating red meat, or had drastically cut their consumption of it.

The importance of nutrition to seniors can hardly be overestimated. Joseph Eastlack, Ph.D., of the Campbell Soup Company, told Dychtwald that "Older people, more aware of their body's frailties than their younger counterparts and fearful of endangering their independent lifestyle, perceive nutrition as a means of promoting good health and resistance to illness."

According to Eastlack, unhealthy foods are increasingly being avoided by seniors; foods that promote health and vitality are increasingly being sought after and consumed.

As early as 1987, a study by Donnelly Marketing found that seniors readily identified cholesterol, salt, calories, and caffeine as the dietary factors they were most concerned about limiting or eliminating altogether, Dychtwald reports.

And while few senior citizens can match 96-year-old Hulda Crooks' claim that "I haven't had a mouthful of meat, fish, or fowl since I was not quite 18," all of the 25 are aware of the benefits of proper nutrition to longevity and the quality of life.

Companionship

The human being is a social animal. One recent study found that, regardless of age, people with strong social bonds—in marriage, or with friends, groups, or organizations—have a 2.4 percent lower mortality rate than those who are isolated.

That, of course, is the ideal. A report by the Reverend Andrew M. Greeley, a sociologist/priest/novelist, claims that the happiest men and women in America are married couples who have sex frequently after the age of 60. Reverend Greeley's report was based on two surveys that involved 5,738 subjects.

Greeley, a sociology professor at the University of Chicago and the University of Arizona, as well as a research associate at The University of Chicago's National Opinion Center, told the Associated Press that men and women who report frequent sex after 60 are more likely to say they are living exciting lives.

Of the men interviewed in *December Champions,* only Phil Guarnaccia was single at the time of the interview. Eighty-year-old Max Rhodes, the wheelchair marathon athlete, married his Japanese translator after a marathon in Japan at age 75. George Bakewell, the 100-year-old softball player, remarried at age *96!*

Unfortunately, life isn't always fair. Many people who have no desire to be single in their later years don't have a choice in the matter. Women simply live longer than men. Dychtwald reports that 60 percent of women over the age of 65 are alone, either through divorce or the loss of a spouse.

Some of the women in *December Champions* live alone, but none of them are lonely. They've found companionship through their involvement in social, civic, and religious activities and/or competition.

It is easy to attribute the incredible rise in participation in Senior Games to a search for companionship as well as a general awareness of physical fitness among seniors. But, interestingly enough, many of the seniors interviewed in *December Champions* credited the practice of "age-grading" (having competitors separated into age brackets: 60–64, 64–69, 70–74, and so on) competitions for their renewed interest.

"It seems that age-graded competitions mean that we end up looking forward to certain birthdays like little kids," Jim Law said. "It is one of the few times that you want to get older.

"I've got a buddy in Charlotte, Jack Wood, who turned 80 in June, 1992. All winter long he was champing at the bit to be 80. His wife said he'd wake up every morning and say, 'Sally, am I 80 yet?' Jack is 80 now and he throws things I can't lift."

Luck

There are just some things that are out of anyone's control. Living to be a vigorous 80 in 1992 means you survived the flu epidemic of 1918–19. It might mean you dodged bullets in World War II. It means you weren't hit by a truck at age 40.

But to run the Ironman Triathlon at 78 involves another kind of luck. You can't help the family you were born into. If you inherited tendencies to diabetes, heart disease, Alzheimer's, cancer, or mental depression, they may limit the extent to which you can become physically fit, though proper exercise and diet afford some protection against some of these.

Still, all else being equal—and Alzheimer's or a piece of shrapnel from Iwo Jima tend to skew the balance—if you take care of yourself, you'll be a December Champion rather than a December Also-Ran.

Richard Sprott, chief researcher for the National Institute on Aging says four things can help a person live longer and better: 1. Buckle your seat belt. 2. Give up smoking. 3. Start a program of regular exercise. 4. Lose some weight if you're overweight.

Dr. Walter Bortz, author of *We Live Too Short and Die Too Long*, adds adequate sleep and rest, and maintaining a sense of humor to that list.

Dr. Mark H. Beers, co-author of *Aging in Good Health*, agrees with the above lists, but adds another two suggestions:

"Be careful about medications. Ask your doctor whether a medication is okay for older people and whether the dose has been adjusted for your age. Be sure that one doctor is aware of all of the medications you take so he or she can check for interactions and other kinds of problems.

"Get a flu shot every fall and a pneumonia vaccine once in a lifetime. Women need annual mammograms and men need annual prostate exams."

In closing, some researchers believe that human life spans will someday expand to 500–600 years *if* the body and mind are cared for.

Knowing all of that—why *not* go ahead and do it now? The National Resource Center on Health Promotion and Aging says that more than half of all people over the age of 65 report no leisure-time physical activity. This probably stems from a lack of knowledge about the benefits of exercise, misconceptions about exercise and aging, and to some degree, a fear of potential injury.

Cardiologist Jerome Fleg, a senior investigator with the National Institute on Aging, says there is no good excuse for not getting physically and mentally fit. "People can gain the fitness benefits of exercise at any age," he said. "There's no cut-off point beyond which you shouldn't exercise."

Go ahead and do it! Whatever it is—a new exercise, a new job, a new hobby, a new friend—*go ahead and do it!*

December Champions is not a collection of quaint stories about cute people doing precocious things. These are 25 stories about 25 dynamic people who are still making a difference. At one point or another, all took control of their lives and challenged the world around them.

They may be "December champions," but they've got a whole new year ahead of them.

Two last pearls of wisdom. Claire Willi, the 100-year-old who was taking a dance class and featured in *Newsweek* had this succinct bit of advice on how to look young at the century mark: "Stand straight—it is very important."

And from actor/comedian/Famous Old Person George Burns, a spry 95: "Don't die. It's been done."

Is not old wine wholesomest, old pippins toothsomest, old wood burn brightest, old linen wash whitest? Old soldiers, sweethearts, are surest, and old lovers are soundest.

—John Webster, "Westward Ho"

Chapter 1

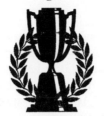

George Bakewell

*In the batter's box, perfect stance, a swing, a dribble, fifty
feet, no more,
Then in flight to first base—that sack is now in right field,
I'm sure.
Oh yes, my friends, the years have rolled by—and I'm not
quite the same,
But thanks be to God, I still enjoy, the playing of the
Grand Old Game.*

—from "Thankful Indeed" by George A. Bakewell

ST. PETERSBURG, FLORIDA—At age 100, George A.
Bakewell is the best-known player on America's best-known
senior softball team, the Kids and Kubs.* They've been featured
on every major television network, in most major magazines,
in more than 200 newspapers, and in a handful of national
commercials.

George himself was spotlighted in a popular 1992
commercial for NIKE shoes. Not only did he get all the best
lines, he took time to put the whole thing in perspective.

"In 1987, I was in a commercial for an insurance man on
the East Coast," George said. "We had a 93-year-old man who
was a bicyclist and a lady who was taking flying lessons—and
she was 102!

"They don't know when to quit nowadays."

The Kids and Kubs' legendary catcher should know a thing
or two about perseverance himself, having been with the team
since 1968.

An only child growing up in Livonia, Michigan, George was
only seven when his mother died. George lived with his father's

sister for three years, until his father remarried.

"He was a farmer and I was a farmer's son," George recalled. "I stayed there on his farm until I was pert' near 24 when I married. The young lady was someone I had known since she was 15 and I was 20. I waited until she was 19.

"We had six children, all of whom are still alive in October 1992, all with their original spouses—285 years of married life among them. I've got 110 on my family tree, including 45 great-grandchildren and six great-great-grandchildren. Isn't that something?"

George played two years of baseball on the town team as a young man before the grandstand burned down. Unfortunately, the grandstand happened to be on some valuable real estate, so they didn't rebuild it.

"Then I got married and baseball became secondary in my life," he said. "We had six youngsters in 12 years—it took most of my time just to keep shoes on their feet! We got married in 1916 and a few years after that was the Great Depression and it was hard going. After I married, I worked for the Ford Motor Co. and I moonlighted in real estate for about 35 years.

"During my time at Ford, I met Mr. Ford and had a conversation with him. His farm and my father's farm were just about eight or nine miles apart. In his younger days, Mr. Ford ran a tractor around the neighborhood. He knew a lot of the people I knew around there because he worked on that tractor and for a lot of farmers.

"One day I ran into Mr. Ford and he said, 'Do you have the little booklet on the sayings of Christ?' I said, 'No.' And he said, 'I'll get you one.'"

The Bakewells moved to Florida in 1950 because of Mrs. Bakewell's failing health.

"In 1967, I tried out for the Kids and Kubs team, but all of the membership was taken up, so I became a batboy," George said. "I got to be a member in 1968 and it was the first time I'd played ball since back in my kid days.

"So I've been with the Kubs 24 years all told—so far. I'm set on being in for my 25th year. There's only been one man who has even reached 20 years besides me, so that's a real honor."

George said that the Kids and Kubs team was founded in 1930 by New York actress Evelyn Barton Rittenhouse as the Three-Quarter Century Softball Club. (The Kids, incidentally, share their St. Petersburg field with the Half-Century Softball Club, which was founded in 1937.)

"I have always taken pride in whatever I've done," he said. "I've been the Kids and Kubs' secretary for 20 years and I'm still the historian. We had a history book for our 44th year, our 50th year, and I'm working on our third for our 64th year. So I've been active with it and I've enjoyed every minute of it. Well, we've had some ups and downs while I've been with the Kids and Kubs, but it has been good for me and I think I've been good for the club."

At the North Shore Park down near Old Tampa Bay,
The Kids and Kubs gather together, a little softball for to play.
This is a tri-weekly event, each and every fall,
These youngsters getting back into shape 'fore the umpire says,
*   "Play ball!"*
To get back in stride, we'll all do our very best indeed,
Boy, oh boy, now using muscles none thought we'd ever need.
Due to our arthritis and lumbago, we're very apt to take
*   a fall,*
But we're up with smiles—all anxious, to hear the umpire
*   say, "Play Ball."*

—from "Play Ball" by George A. Bakewell

The Kids and Kubs play a full schedule. The 1992 program listed a tour through Pennsylvania in July, and the Senior Softball World Series near Detroit. Additionally, the Kubs had a full slate of charity games scheduled from December 1992, to March 1993, against teams representing the Salvation Army, Goodwill Industries, local schools, and other teams and organizations.

"Right now I can play four innings without any trouble at all," George said. "I don't have any trouble breathing, because my lungs are wonderful. As everybody knows, your legs give out first. So my only trouble has been because—as everybody also knows—they keep moving that first base sack further and further out into right field with each year!

"I hit the ball hard enough. Anything above my knees, I'm pretty good at determining the strike zone. I haven't struck out swinging in two years. I *have* been called out on strikes, especially if the ball is below the knees. That may be because I have cataracts on both eyes. If it gets down near the ground, I can't tell the distance."

George passed on the trip to Michigan in 1992, and, out of

102 teams, the Kubs managed to make the semifinals without him. He said he's cutting back on some of the longer out-of-town trips to let younger players get some more playing time.

"One trip I remember especially well was the team's trip to Sacramento and I got to take my wife along," George said. "I remarried when I was 96, and my wife Bonnie and I went to Sacramento with the team.

"But on this team, every day is a special day and every day is a little different. During the course of a season, we usually lose an average of 3.4 men to death or retirement, partly because you can't start playing until you're in your 75th year.

"But the Kids and Kubs still play to win."

But there is more to the Kids and Kubs than what happens between the foul lines. In addition to being the club's secretary and historian, George is currently serving as its director emeritus. He says the Kubs didn't always have the prosperity they now enjoy.

"In the early '70s, I was still a secretary in the club and we got down to $16.61 in the treasury," he said. "So the president of the club and I went down Central Avenue here and sold $750 in advertisements and that's as near as we ever got to being broke.

"Right now we've got about $70,000 in a trust fund and the interest is $500 per month. We've got another fund that supports that and we get the interest. We've got $70,000 all in good bonds and so forth.

"Each year the Kids and Kubs also print up a brochure that has our lineup and something about our history. It's not much, but it does have some advertisements and raises some money for us."

You don't maintain George's kind of schedule—on and off the field—if you're not physically fit. George said that he has been exercising regularly for the past 25 of his 100 years.

"My wife was sick for 64 days once and the doctor said, 'I don't know if it is contagious or not, George—but you need to take care of your wife. I don't think it's serious, but I don't want to take any chances. I want you to get in shape so you can take care of her.'

"So I learned to do exercises then and I've been exercising ever since. I work at climbing stairs and I've got a pipe here that's 42 inches long and weighs six pounds and I lift it 50 times per day.

"You can't figure, 'Well, next week I'm going to do this or that.' You can't prepare for it all in one day because it doesn't happen that way. I try to keep in shape."

Staying in shape is a continual process. He recommends that people look for ways to increase their flexibility and endurance in the little things they do in their everyday lives.

"Don't just walk across the floor, tiptoe once in a while," he said. "It's true that the legs give out first. I've got good legs, yeah. And I was at the doctor's for an examination yesterday and he took my blood pressure and it was 152/80. The doctor said, 'George, that's perfect for your age.'

"In the last few years, the only time I've seen doctors was when I was 85 and had a prostate gland operation and two years ago when I had diverticulitis. I see two specialists every three months or so, and I have a family doctor I see every once in a while or when I feel like it. The last three exams have been perfect. In fact, they've said, 'You're getting better with age, George.'"

Like many seniors, George says that, in addition to exercise, he attributes his longevity to careful eating habits.

"I never was a heavy eater, and I never liked fatty foods of any kind, and I never cared for fried foods," he said. "I eat what I want to eat. I'm not picky or choosy wherever I go—I join right in with them. I am a light eater. I eat plenty of vegetables and fruit. I'm not much of a meat-eater, although I like gravy. But not meat. My weight is always around 142 pounds.

"One thing I noticed: you can tell the steady smokers on the team. I watch them passing out before they hit 80! I never smoked, I never drank, so that's a plus.

> *When out on the field we sure enough all like to let it go,*
> *The spirit may be willing, but the flesh oftentimes says no.*
> *We're all young at heart, never count the birthdays at all,*
> *The years are soon forgotten when the umpire says,*
> *"Play ball!"*

> —"Play Ball" by George A. Bakewell

George said that he's planning a full schedule in 1993, but may taper off in the future. He wants "younger thoughts" to take over his position as historian. ("I've got the material for it, but I'll let someone else put it together.") And he thinks it is time for him to play fewer games, in part because he believes his new-found notoriety is taking attention away from the Kids and Kubs.

Much of that attention has come following his appearance on a '92 television ad for NIKE shoes.

"This series on NIKE began in April 1992," he said. "They came with four big vans of traveling gear. I was at the ballpark from 8 a.m. to 2 p.m. Then on the 7th of July, a man took my wife and me over to Tampa, where they asked me questions for the cameras. That advertisement cost $120,000 for 30 seconds. And when they got through checking me out, they'd do things like ask me how old Babe Ruth would be if he were alive today? And I'd say, 'If the Babe were alive, he'd be two years older than me.' Then they'd say, 'That took a second too long,' and we'd do it again.

"Then there was the thing I said at the end: 'Perhaps it's your shoes.' Well, I didn't know what that meant. That went right over my head."

Since then, George said he has been inundated with calls and proposals for additional appearances and interviews.

"NIKE invited my wife and me to San Diego to see the All-Star Game, all expenses paid," he said. "Since I got back, the phones have kept ringing and I've got a list of 18 TV and radio stations that have contacted me, from California to Iowa to New York.

"Just recently I got a call from NBC—they'll be down in a week or so. And both 'Entertainment Tonight' and CBS in New York have called and said they're going to do special programs for late '92."

Actually, George said he's only seen the NIKE commercial once.

"I get tired of watching a ballgame that takes more than two hours to play," he said. "Back in my day, if you didn't get done in two hours, there was something wrong! I think it's because of the commercials."

Don't tell NIKE.

For George, making the commercial was interesting, but he wouldn't consider it a highlight in his life. He says what matters more is when he can make a change in someone's life.

"I've had two mothers in the last 10 years come up to me and say, 'I want to introduce my boys to you and I want you to tell them a little lesson,'" George said. "When that happens, I say, 'Boys, if you want to live and play ball at my age, you don't smoke and you don't drink. You learn to say no.'

"Maybe the kids laugh at you. Or maybe they'll see you play and say, 'Well, he's all right.' The last time I checked over on these boys, they were doing just that. They were saying no. If I can save just one boy from doing wrong, I've done pretty good."

Somebody must agree. When George turned 100 in April 1992, family and friends from across the United States and from as far away as Germany came to attend the ceremony.

"We had 180 in the church—that's quite a crowd!" he said.

He says he has had a wonderful life and gives credit to "three wonderful women:

"My mother—she died when I was seven; my first wife—we were married for sixty-five and one-half years, and my second wife. We married on my 96th birthday and we've had a wonderful time. For our wedding trip, one of my boys took us on a trip to Switzerland. We've also been to San Diego and Sacramento, and we've had some wonderful trips together.

"I consider myself an optimistic person and I still think there is Somebody bigger than you and me here, too. I've been a church member all my life and I still have my beliefs. I don't think I could do this whole thing myself."

George says there is more to his life than just baseball. He stays actively involved in his giant extended family. He writes a little poetry. He speaks to civic and service organizations when asked.

"I hope to be here another 10 years—I'm shooting for the year 2000," he said. "I see no reason, barring an accident... I'm in good shape, I've got three doctors watching me and they're all very good, very thorough—and I like it that way. I like to be checked up every three months in case anything should happen, because I am an old man. At the same time, I've been very, very lucky all my life."

From the above you know of fun and excitement, I've had my
  full share;
Still endowed by a host of kind friends who really, really care.
While going through this span of years, I picked up a habit I enjoy,
  I must say,
I'm known as The Kissing Bandit—one kiss, then: "George,
  you've really made my day!"

—from "Birth to 100 Years" by George A. Bakewell

Now as we travel life's pathways 'mid this earthly strife
and woe,
Let's do our best to scatter a little sunshine wherever we
doth go.
When our 'Book of Life' is closed and we answer the
Master's call,
May we all be ready and willing when our 'Umpire in
Chief' says, "Play ball!"

—from "Play Ball" by George A. Bakewell

---

* The Kids and Kubs bill themselves as: "The Granddaddy of All Softball Teams. St. Petersburg's Greatest Publicity Asset since 1931 (next to sunshine)."

Chapter 2

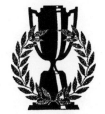

Ken Beer

HILLSBOROUGH, CALIFORNIA—Eighty-nine-year-old Ken Beer is the Babe Ruth, Jim Brown, and Jack Nicklaus of senior tennis all rolled into one. He's dominated the Senior 80 Singles as few athletes have ever dominated their sport.

Through mid-1992, Ken has won more than 70 major tournaments, including the Senior 80 Singles five times, the Men's 85 National Grass Court Championship Singles four times, the Men's 85 National Indoor Championships three times, and the Men's 85 National Clay Court Championships two times—all since 1983! (He's also won the 85 doubles in these various tournaments numerous times, usually with Ferd Kramer or Herbert Hauser.)

Next year he goes into the Senior 90 division and it'll be "Katy bar the door!" for Ken Beer! After playing men seven, eight, even nine years his junior in tournaments in recent years, Ken says he's ready to blaze new ground.

Actually, the Beers have always been pioneers of some sort. Both of his parents were early settlers in Utah. Ken's grandmother walked across the Great Plains in 1862 at age 16!

Ken grew up in Salt Lake City, attended high school there, and eventually was graduated from Stanford University. In 1927, he joined the Army Air Corps. Three years later he was hired by Pan Am, where he remained until he retired in 1963 at age 60.

During World War II, Ken was in charge of both pilot training and Pan Am's civilian transport with U.S. government operations in the Pacific theater.

"I was flying the Pacific with Pan Am when the United States took over my division en masse," Ken said, "but they didn't do anything different except to tell us what to take and where to take it. So that's what we did. We operated under the auspices of the Navy, but we retained our unit as it had been during peacetime.

"I was based in San Francisco, but I flew all over the Pacific. We didn't get close to the battlefields because we were only carrying personnel and equipment, so they didn't want us to be in the firing line. We still went fairly close and, when the South Pacific was pretty hot, we went into Australia. And as they moved north, we moved into some of the more northern islands and eventually got back to the Philippines.

"I hit mandatory retirement at age 60. (I know it's the law, but I was as sound then as ever and the law is wrong.)"

Before retirement, Ken was Pan Am's senior pilot, known for both his jaunty air and his ever-present tennis racket. From about age 30 on, "social" tennis has been his passion.

"I used to carry my racket wherever I flew," he said. "Mainly for exercise after flying. I found it was the best antidote for flying fatigue. So I played it regularly and some places I met tennis players and some places some of my copilots/pilots were tennis players as well. So I got plenty of exercise that way.

"I played all over the Pacific: Bangkok, Hong Kong, Guam, the South Pacific, wherever I could play. I thoroughly enjoyed it. I met some nice people, got invited to some nice clubs. So it served a dual purpose. I played Tokyo Tennis Club where the emperor of Japan plays—and, although I didn't play with him, that's where all of the best tennis players in Tokyo played. I played in Manila at the Manila Tennis Club, where several world champions played."

He also became something of a connoisseur of tennis courts along the way.

"From a scenic standpoint, Hong Kong was probably the most spectacular," he said. "The city of Hong Kong is on the main island and across the bay is the mainland with Kowloon. I found it fascinating. Of course, it has a history that goes back hundreds of years. I thoroughly enjoyed Hong Kong.

"I enjoyed Bangkok, too. It was very peaceful the time we were there and we were there during the early days of flying. We were still somewhat of a novelty back then. So much so that the bus that would bring the crew through the center of town would attract the attention of the people riding the little tricycle-type vehicles called 'samlo'—which means three wheels. They used to wave to us. We got quite friendly with a number of them.

"They were a quiet, friendly people and Bangkok was especially interesting. The people were so interesting, the area was so interesting—because it is very much like Venice, full of canals."

Beer made one more epic journey in his flying career. In aviation record books there is a notation for Capt. Kenneth V. Beer. On November 18, 1946, Ken piloted the Pan-American clipper Golden West from Honolulu to Los Angeles—a distance of 2,550 miles—in the record-breaking time of eight hours and 54 minutes. Ken's giant flying boat bested the previous record by five minutes.

After retirement, Ken considered, for the first time, playing something other than friendly tennis.

"I picked up competitive tennis at age 60 because I enjoyed the game immensely," he said. "I've always had a lot of fun playing tennis, and since I did well, I've kept it up. I haven't shied away from other sports, I just got into tennis and stayed with it. I've always skied and swum a lot. But since I've played social tennis since I was 30, the transition at age 60 to competitive tennis was only a matter of travel."

Friends and family convinced him to enter his first National Super Seniors Tennis Tournament in Florida in 1964, and he's been participating in tournament tennis ever since. And since 1964, he's won a *lot* of those tennis tournaments.

"Through spring of 1992, I've won 70 national tournaments," he said, with just a hint of justifiable pride in his voice. "Of those championships, the thing that stands out most in my memory are the tournaments I didn't win! I remember the losses. The losses educate me, they help to correct what I'm doing wrong, they show me what to work on. Whenever I'd lose to someone, I'd have to get in there and find out why! That's what I remember about those tournaments—the ones I didn't win.

"That reflects my outlook on life. I believe losses set parameters on your education. In winning, the climax is successful, but you really don't learn too much from winning. You learn more from losing. A lot of people don't realize that losing is very educational because it tells you what you can't do and that helps you to grow."

Education has a price, of course, and it is a price that Ken Beer is willing to pay. Take May 1992, for example. That month, Ken participated in four tournaments: two local and two national (the nationals were the National Hardcourt

Tournament in Santa Barbara, California, and the Indoor Championships in Boise, Idaho). It was a schedule that would tax a man half his age.

"I won the singles division in all four of them, and won the doubles title in Boise," he said. "We shouldn't have lost the doubles title in Santa Barbara, but they played both championships on the same day. After five and a half hours of tennis in one day, I was a little tired!"

Ken's favorite stop in the Super Seniors is the Longwood Cricket Club in Chestnut Hill, Massachusetts. Many of the tournaments he's won have been at Longwood, which is the unofficial "home" of seniors tennis.

"Next year I get to play in the Men's 90s bracket," he said. "Unfortunately, there are only half a dozen good 90-year-old tennis players in the United States at the moment. Well, there's one old boy in Maine who beat me in 1991, who gives me some pretty good competition, but I beat him this year."

The caliber of his competition is something that Ken is deadly serious about.

"I prefer to play people who are at least a little better than I am," he said. "It makes me work. I have an engagement tonight to play team tennis at our club. I'll be up against players who are 30–40 years younger than I am. I don't know how I'll do, but I'll go up against them because that's how you get better.

"Earlier today I got beaten by someone 10 years younger. Of course, at our club, I often play with members who are 20–30 years younger. I'll play anybody who asks me and I will ask people to play who are my equal, or just a little behind me. It's not polite to ask people who are better than you are to play. They should ask you first."

Ken's stamina and skill at his age are inspiring even to non-tennis players. He has a wicked backhand, seems to run effortlessly, and has a surprising amount of power for a man who is only a thin, wiry 5'6" tall. He claims to follow no special diet, save that he's always eaten in moderation. And if you didn't know he was 89, you wouldn't think his daily workout is particularly demanding, either.

"I don't have a formal daily exercise routine," he said. "I keep doing everything I can. I have a philosophy that, if something gets hard, just do it! If you keep giving up on the hard things, of course, you keep giving up on more and more things as you get older. So I subscribe to the opposite: if it is difficult to do, do it.

"I've also swum a great deal in my life. I used to swim at all the islands we flew to, of course! But I don't swim as much as I used to because I spend more of my time playing tennis. I try to play tennis almost every day. Things will come up and I can't do it—certain obligations around the house, whatever. But there are very few weeks that I don't play at least six times.

"As for my physical fitness now, I have no complaints. I get tired quicker now than I used to. I can play three–four hours without getting tired, but *boy* I'll show it the next day. I've always been fairly injury-free. Well, I severed an Achilles tendon skiing 15 years ago, but it healed so well I now forget which leg it was!"

Interestingly enough, Ken says that his personal physicians have expressed mixed feelings about such a strenuous level of activity for a man born in 1903.

"My doctors argue and disagree heartily with me all the time about everything I do, especially tennis," Ken said with a laugh. "They say, 'Well, which medical college did *you* graduate from?' I say, 'Pal, I graduated with a million years of human experience!' Most of them don't have much of a leg to stand on because while I'm aged 89, they're all in worse shape than me! It is impossible to talk me out of it.

"Now I will say I've got one doctor friend who is a good tennis player. He's 30 years younger and he's supportive of my playing tennis. Someday I'm going to beat him, too. I keep telling him, 'You're getting older; someday my day will come.'"

Don't bet against Ken, either.

In the meantime, his exploits on the tennis court have spawned dozens of magazine and newspaper write-ups. He's achieved something of a hero status both in his hometown of Hillsborough and at the Longwood Cricket Club.

"More than anything else, I think, because the media want something to fill up the space, rather than because of anything I've done," he said. "I have had a few bits of publicity. I don't find publicity annoying or anything, I just take it for what it's worth. People who are interested in pursuing that type of activity, that's fine. I don't resist, but I don't overemphasize it, either. I feel I'm just plain lucky, so I'm not going to trade on it. I take publicity very lightly.

"You see, I figure that I'm fortunate. People are always asking me, 'How do you live so long and still work?' I say, 'You pick the right parents!' I'd say 90 percent of my success is through luck. So I take it as it is. I don't trade on it."

That modest attitude, coupled with his prodigious achievements, have made Ken Beer a popular speaker and a favorite at any tournament in which he competes. Those who know him say he perpetually looks on the bright side of life, another trait that endears him to tennis players, young and old alike.

"I do try to look on the good side of things," he said. "If I've got work to do, I recognize that work is good for me and I just pitch in and do it. I welcome any exercise, any stretching that comes with it. Sure, I look on the pleasant side of anything. Why make life hard on yourself?

"Well, my children call me a Pollyanna. I try to be a realist; I just don't look on the sad side of life."

Consequently, he's often mobbed at tournaments by players wanting advice, friends wanting to get re-acquainted, and people of all ages wanting to know where he found the Fountain of Youth.

"When someone asks, 'How long can I play tennis?' I say, 'Just keep playing and find out.' A lot of people can go into their 90s and keep playing well. You just have to keep on playing.

"And for a young person who wants to be this active at age 90, I say pick out what you want to do and go after it wholeheartedly. Do the thing you like the best—and it doesn't matter what it is—and that's the way you'll succeed."

There is much more to Ken Beer than winning tennis tournaments and doing magazine interviews. Ken and his wife Mavia have four children, including a daughter who is a top-ranked tennis player in California.

And Ken is still an active participant in the learning process. A conversation with Ken might range from the monkey worship in Thailand to ancient religions—"When you see the philosophies that have underpinned Chinese or Egyptian civilizations for 6,000 years, you know you can learn something from them!"—to the demise of his beloved Pan Am. He reads avidly, everything from physics to astronomy. He considers himself a nature worshipper, an environmentalist, and a naturalist—who just happens to be, pound for pound, year for year, the best tennis player on the planet.

"If something comes along that I haven't succeeded at—then, great!" he said. "That's something new to plow into!"

Chapter 3

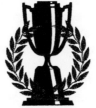

Edward Bishop

SAN FRANCISCO, CALIFORNIA—San Francisco Bay is cold and crowded, turbulent and treacherous. The wind howls in from the north and west even in the summer, tossing whitecaps and sea gulls before it, swirling around the rocks, howling through the bridges. It is there that you'll find 71-year-old Edward Bishop windsurfing. It is there that you'll find Edward Bishop following the wind.

Another day you may find him windsurfing amid the placid waters of Lake Merced. Still another may find him daring Maui's beautiful but challenging waves.

For Edward Bishop, windsurfing is like a quest.

"The wind and water have always been quite special to me," he said. "They have almost a spiritual quality. Being out in the wind and on the water is a very, very special experience that I find hard to put into words. It is an almost spiritual awareness under those conditions. I can completely forget almost anything when I'm concentrating on the wind and waves.

"Since my time as a navigator with the Royal Air Force, watching the wind and weather has fascinated me. Windsurfing enables me to do it in a comfortable way—but one I am intimately connected with. I feel that's a valuable experience."

Edward was born in England, the son of religious parents who were active in missions in the East End of London. He attended Leyton County High School for Boys where he was active in gymnastics, European handball, soccer—even American baseball.

"I never went to college," he recalled in his still-crisp British accent. "I obtained a scholarship to study agriculture. With it, I was required to work on a farm to gain experience, since I'd been brought up as a city kid.

"I decided to work the second year on a farm, but then the war came in 1939 and I volunteered for the Royal Air Force (RAF) in 1940. I qualified as a wireless operator and a tail gunner. Then I became a navigator."

In short order, the RAF switched from three-man crews to two-man crews and Edward was quickly certified as a navigator as well. As a member of the transport command, he completed three tours in North Africa and the Middle East.

"One of my more interesting commitments came when I was attached to two American squadrons because they had to fly their fighters from England down into Italy and support the advance there. But they had radar operators aboard who had no navigation experience," he said. "So my pilot and I were attached to these two squadrons for six weeks to give them training. After that, I decided that that was too big a commitment—the normal navigator training is six months! But I led them out to Gibralter and North Africa in formation."

A bout with amoebic dysentery ended the war for Edward and he was shipped back to Britain where he worked first as an X-ray technician and later, as an X-ray engineer ("because there seemed to be more money in that.") When the National Health Service was instituted in 1948, socialized medicine ended *that* career as well.

"So I emigrated to Canada," he said. "I'd done a lot of work, developmental and experimental work, with animals at the Royal Veterinary College just outside London, and tried to follow this up. And after a few wanderings again, I ended up at the Ontario Veterinary College, in charge of their X-ray department.

"Once there I was able to develop new ideas for the study of animals. Up until that time, a lot of work had been done on animals, but only as experimental work for human benefit. Whereas I was able to turn it backwards and work mainly for the benefit of animals. I was able to develop a number of pieces of equipment which made it much easier to work with animals, from chinchillas to horses."

Within a few years, Edward was lecturing fourth-year veterinary students in radiology and conducting clinical sessions for the fifth-year students—all without the benefit of a degree.

But after seven years, a change in the administration ended yet another opportunity.

"One pharmaceutical company had given me a lot of material for some work I'd done on dogs' lungs and on kennel cough," he said. "I was able to demonstrate that dogs get a lot of conditions also recognized in humans.

"So the company offered me the chance to go to western Canada as a detail man or pharmaceutical representative. That worked out very well, and over the years I became sales executive for western Canada. I covered the far western part of the system. Then I went back to Toronto as assistant to the national sales and advertising sales manager."

When not out selling or developing advertising campaigns, Edward was busy snow- and water-skiing, sailing, and playing badminton and table tennis. He also operated a store in Kingston, Ontario, that sold fine nautical equipment and accessories.

"I had become very involved and interested in sailing," he said. "When I heard that the 1976 Olympics were going to be in Montreal and that the sailing site would probably be in Kingston, I went there and opened this store and joined the local yacht club. I managed to get to be one of the people who drove the spectator control and support boats at the Olympics.

"So for six weeks in the pre-Olympic year and the Olympic year, I was out sailing and observing some of the best sailors in the world. I was very fortunate that the people at the Kingston Yacht Club were very keen and very knowledgeable sailors. They knew how to set courses in the Atlantic racing affairs— which was one reason Kingston was chosen as the Olympic sailing site."

After the Olympics, Edward was hopelessly hooked on sailing. He sailed competitively for nearly 13 years in a number of boats, including a 28-foot Viking, a number of CNC-27s, and—most importantly—in Sharks.

"Sharks have a three-man crew and they can sail under just about any conditions," he said. "Our crew was very successful. One year we came in 10th or 11th in the American competition, and 22nd in the Shark World Competition. It was rather satisfying."

About this time, Edward also began working as a volunteer in something similar to what is known as a hospice in the United States—called Parenting Care—in Canada. He counseled and consoled people who were dying, as well as their relatives. It was enormously rewarding work, but draining emotionally and spiritually.

"I did this for eight to 10 years before I decided I needed a rest and went back to sailing," he said. "But rather than get involved with a crew, I decided to try windsurfing. This was about 1985.

"I had a friend who had a board and I went to watch him. It looked very easy so I decided to have a go. I was sufficiently successful to be really attracted. I still spent a very trying, very frustrating four months trying to master the basic essentials without being very good at it."

Finally, Edward swallowed his pride and began to take lessons from an instructor who worked out of Kingston on Lake Ontario.

"Lake Ontario is about 40 miles wide in places and 200 miles long and has some quite heavy weather," he said. "When I could stand on the wretched thing and handle the wind, the waves would come and knock me down. And when I was able to handle the waves, the wind would blow me over.

"So I had a rather frustrating period, which I worked through. I found ways to get around and found windsurfing an absolutely fascinating experience."

There were other changes afoot in Edward's life. After an amiable divorce, he met an American lady in New York, got married, and ultimately settled with his new wife in San Francisco.

"When I came to California," Edward said, "I went to rent a board and the man I rented from said, 'You know, you would make a good instructor. You should take the instructor's course.' I thought that was quite ridiculous. But he said, 'No, come on! You'd be quite good at it!' He was remarkably supportive, but he was also firm and he pushed me to improve my skills in the instructor's course.

"I'm certainly not an outstanding wave jumper or anything like that, but I enjoy windsurfing, and during the last two years I've really enjoyed teaching.

"I've found with most students with whom I work, I can cut the agonizing four-month period I went through to sometimes four hours—or, at most, two days. With the teaching methods we have now, it's rare when we don't get people going in two days. It is very satisfying to start with. There are some people who are kind of overweight or who are not very strong or are apprehensive in the water, and they really glow and get a great deal of satisfaction out of learning to windsurf successfully."

In fact, Edward has grown to love teaching windsurfing so much that he's never been intrigued by the growing Masters

Windsurfing competitions that are springing up around the country.

"My wife tells me I'm not very sensible in a lot of things, but I know that at 71, I do have some physical limitations," he said. "I'm not at the level of skill (as far as I know), to compete."

That hasn't prevented Edward from becoming a popular and much-in-demand windsurfing instructor in the Bay Area. While the majority of his students are in their 20s and 30s, he says he's had a few people in their 50s learn to windsurf. But none, to date, in their 70s.

"I enjoy windsurfing as a sport and I encourage other people to enjoy the satisfaction of being up on a board, and the thrill of speed, and getting out in the open air," he said.

"And I've taught some people who were very overweight. That was quite demanding in things like finding the right equipment—and it's almost as big a problem with people who are very underweight. It takes a little careful thought to find equipment that is right for the individual.

"Every day is very different, with different challenges."

The hunt for new challenges has taken Edward and his board up and down the West Coast and beyond.

"I particularly enjoy windsurfing on Lake Merced because of the delightful scenery surrounding it," he said.

"But of the places that are the most special to me, Maui in Hawaii is one of those, although I was rather disappointed in my own accomplishments in windsurfing there.

"I went to Hawaii in the Christmas of 1991, and every time I went out, I had to be rescued. I just wiped out. The winds were high and the water was rough and, in my childish enthusiasm, I wiped out each time. I did learn an awful lot about self-rescue and survival, and I was able get back up in one piece and go out the next day."

For all of his exploits, Edward fancies himself an "undramatic, somewhat dull visitor."

"I just enjoy doing things," he said. "I usually expect things to go wrong, so I'm not usually surprised when they do. Looking back on it now, I've told a few people my story about the aircraft I crashed in during the war—which is a fairly normal procedure—and they find it incredible.

"I find a lot things don't impress me as dangerous. I've enjoyed white-water rafting, a little hang gliding. I've done the things I've just wanted to do. They don't have a sort of exceptional quality... to me."

Maybe not to Edward, but his list of accomplishments sound pretty impressive to most under-70 landlubbers and lay people. He admits, however, that he would not be able to undertake all of those strenuous activities unless he kept his 71-year-old body in shape through exercise and a proper diet.

"I do a number of what we used to call calisthenics every morning on my own and I feel much better when I do," he said. "And I do walk a fair amount.

"My diet tends to be largely, but not strictly, vegetarian. I eat virtually no red meat. This was mainly through the encouragement of my daughter, who was very concerned about the amount of natural resources needed to produce meat. So I've tended towards fruit and vegetables and I enjoy them very much. I do eat poultry and a lot of fish, but I would say that I have a fairly healthy diet with lots of bulk and lots of fiber."

Edward's interest in fitness has carried over into other facets of his life. He currently works with an organization called the Coalition of Agencies Serving the Elderly.

"One of the things we organize is a walk in Golden Gate Park for seniors each September," he said. "We have 3,000 seniors enjoy that walk. I'm also working to organize a walking association in the Bay Area."

One of his other interests harkens back to his veterinary days. Edward works with the legendary gorillas Koko and Michael. Koko is the famous ape that has been taught sign language and once adopted a kitten. Koko's story has been immortalized in the best-selling children's book, *Koko's Kitten*.

"The keepers were kind enough to give me the opportunity to work with them, so I've studied sign language, and I've found that to be a remarkable experience. I'm quite handy with tools and I've helped build a number of partitions and bits and pieces for the animals.

"One of the things I really enjoy is working out ways to do things. There is an awful lot of improvising at the hospital, including finding new ways to work with old equipment. While at the veterinary college, I developed a lot of things. So I've continued to work towards finding ways to achieve things that haven't been done before.

"I have another invention in the process that could be a way of dividing people into safe spaces during earthquakes or other natural disasters. I just enjoy looking at problems and finding ways to get around them."

Fortunately, for a man whose interests range from

windsurfing to talking with gorillas, Edward's family has encouraged his various activities.

"My children have been extremely supportive," he said. "Sometimes a little surprised, though!

"My wife joins me in most of the things I do, except that she doesn't like windsurfing, she likes boogie boarding—and I don't like that, so we separate on that, but we enjoy many other things together."

One question that's frequently asked as Edward teaches windsurfing is, "Can I really do what you're still doing when I reach age 71?"

"I see a lot of people who suddenly say, 'Oh, I reached the big 50 or 60—I can't do things anymore,'" he said. "Which I think is just ridiculous. I think if people tell themselves they can't, they *won't* be able to do something. If they tell themselves they can, they probably can. Look around and you'll see a lot of overweight people in their 20s and 30s. If they want to remain active, they certainly can, and they can enjoy it.

"I was fortunate in being in the Royal Air Force in my 20s in that the atmosphere there was to be fit. We were also fortunate in that the permanent RAF stations had gymnasiums and squash courts. I enjoyed horseback riding, too, and kept that up throughout my life.

"So I say: 'Watch your diet, eat sensibly, be moderate, and if you want to have a drink, have a drink. And if you feel like having a go at something, then have a go! Give it a try. The worst thing you can do is fail. But you may be greatly surprised to find out that you've succeeded.'"

Of course, Edward cautions listeners that *any* new exercise or sport needs to be preceded by some common-sense precautions and preliminaries.

"Now, if you are going to take up something, like a new sport, prepare yourself for it a little beforehand," he said. "Stretch your back, bend your legs and knees, stretch your arms—if there is going to be something involving upper-body strength— and recognize the fact that you're *not* a teen-ager anymore, that you may have to approach it a little more slowly. But the chances are that you'll approach it with more dedication because you're really committed to it.

"Certainly, when I teach people windsurfing, one of the things I really work on is building up their confidence and enthusiasm in themselves. It is surprising the number of people who don't have that, who go through life fearful all the time."

He said this is much the same advice that he gives older people interested in turning their lives around.

"I would say: Watch yourself. You're not going to be able to leap off a galloping horse or a motorcycle. But there are still a lot of things you can do very well. You might be very surprised at how much you can attain.

"I was watching the 1992 U.S. Open recently—I haven't played very much tennis because I wrecked my right shoulder and right elbow playing soccer—but I found that, if you go for all of the shots, even though they may look pretty well impossible, you'll hit a surprising number back.

"I think in a lot of situations, it is an attitude of 'Have a go at it.' For one period in my life I was known as 'Have-a-Go Bishop' because I'd say, 'Let's have a go at anything that comes along.'"

So, what *is* next for "Have-a-Go" Bishop?

"I don't think about a long way down the road, because I recognize that I'm 71," he said. "On the other hand, I plan quite carefully. When I trained salesmen, I emphasized the importance of budgeting time as much as budgeting money, and I've tried to carry that out myself. I like to know the night before what I'm going to be doing the next day so I can adjust my dress to whatever I'm going to do.

"So I like to plan my schedule ideally a year or so ahead. Twenty years ahead I'm not worried about. I do like to know what I'm going to do next month or six months from now."

One thing you can bet on is that next month, six months, even years from now, you'll find him spending every spare minute on some sizable body of water, enjoying the feel of the wind and the spray on his face.

For Edward Bishop, it doesn't get much better than this.

"Windsurfing appeals to me on several levels," he said. "I really love messing around the water, and windsurfing one can do relatively inexpensively. The equipment is specialized, but it is easy to transport and to deal with. Once you've got over the basics, you can enjoy it quite quickly.

"Additionally, I meet some delightful people. Most windsurfers are very open, very sociable and friendly—a very nice community—so that windsurfing really meets many of my needs and interests."

If they're all like Edward Bishop, they're bound to be an exceptional lot, indeed.

Chapter 4

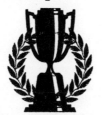

"Banana" George Blair

WINTER HAVEN, FLORIDA—Captain's log, Whaler's Bay, Antarctica, Summer 1986, water temperature—28 degrees:

"Today, we met our first iceberg, saw our first humpback whale... and Mr. George Blair performed his barefoot water-skiing along the beach."

With that notable feat, "Banana" George Alfred Blair became the first person to water-ski—barefoot or otherwise—on or off all seven continents.

And that's only *one* of his spectacular accomplishments. The 77-year-old is a self-made millionaire, a member of the Water Ski Hall of Fame, a featured attraction at Cypress Gardens, star of his own Armor All commercial, world-champion water-skier in a number of age divisions and skill categories, 11-time American barefoot water-ski champion, noted philanthropist, and banana-fanatic.

Did we mention the color yellow? George's homes in New Jersey, Paris, Winter Haven, New York City, and elsewhere are positively *glowing* with yellow. His lemon-yellow speedboat has a reported 400 gold-plated parts. His home telephones are banana-shaped and yellow. His two Cadillacs—the ones he's seen polishing in his Armor All commercial—are yellow. His wet suit and skis are even yellow.

And, each Christmas at Cypress Gardens, he wears a yellow Santa suit and gives out gifts. His name? *Banana Claus.*

"Yellow has been a lifelong passion," George said between performances at Cypress Gardens. "People ask, 'Why do you like yellow?' I say, 'God gave me this thing, I don't know why.'

"That's what I told David Letterman when we were on the tube having our little chat. I said, 'Do you have a favorite color, Mr. Letterman?' He said, 'Well, I guess my favorite color is blue. I guess they ought to call me Mr. Grape or Mr. Blueberry.' So we had a little fun with that but it's the truth. It just comes naturally with me that if I see anything yellow, I'm attracted to it."

What's amazing is that George Blair's life has *always* been this interesting. He's overcome poverty and two potentially paralyzing accidents to water-ski his way into near-legendary status in this country and abroad.

After all, how many other 77-year-olds get sent two *tons* of free bananas each year from Chiquita Brands, *and* can barefoot ski while holding the rope with their teeth?

George's Ohio childhood was pleasant but uneventful. His father played a few sports for fun and one of his brothers ran cross-country in college. In grade school and junior high, George participated in the Junior Olympics at the city of Toledo, and won a few track events in the city-wide competition. To the best of his recollection, he *did* wear shoes for each event.

In high school, golfing became his passion. George was a four-year letterman on the golf team and captain for three of those years.

"One year I was runner-up to the junior champion of the state of Ohio," he said, "only because my father built a golf course. As a matter of fact, he built two of them—and I played a lot. I played every day in the summer and I played fast and hard. I would play 18 holes in two hours—now it takes them five hours to play 18 holes. I couldn't wait to hit the next ball and make it better than the one before, or to get closer to the green on the next shot. I was playing nearly scratch golf when I was a sophomore in high school. But that was only because I played, played, played like crazy because I loved the game."

His other passion was ice skating. And like golf, he participated in it the only way he knew how: full-tilt.

"I *loved* to ice skate," George said. "I was in seventh heaven when I was on racing blades. I would be out on the ice just stroking it as hard as I could stroke it, going as fast as I could. It didn't matter how many friends I had along or no friends— I was just like a bird on the ice. Sometimes I would jump obstacles, like barrels. And sometimes I'd fall and, of course, it would always be on the base of my spine."

But, as happened to so many upper-middle-class families, the Great Depression destroyed the Blair family fortune, all but ending his golfing and ice-skating days.

"We were on easy street, everything we wanted was ours,"

George recalled. "But the Crash and the subsequent real estate depression ended that. My father was in real estate and he lost everything, my uncle lost everything, even my grandfather lost everything. The whole family was destitute overnight. So I went to college without any funds from my family. I worked my way through Miami of Ohio."

During George's sophomore year at Miami, his friends decided to go to Fort Lauderdale for Easter. Despite not having any money, George decided to go, too. The next day he hopped a freight train for Florida.

"In 1934, I officially became a hobo," he said. "So here I was on this freight car with nothing but a can of beans. Unfortunately, there were two other hobos on the same freight car, and when they saw my can of beans, they came over and wanted it. When I said I was not about to give it to them because I didn't have any more cans or money, they picked me up by my arms and my legs and threw me off the freight train going about 30 miles per hour! I landed on my spine. Again."

George's back never fully recovered.

"For years, the only way I could get out of bed each morning was to fall out of bed on my hands and knees, and then slowly creep to the wall and pull myself up by holding on to a wash basin or something like that, and then slowly getting my spine eased into decent condition," he said. "And sometimes the pain would be so great that my wife JoAnne would have to hold me upside down so I could stand on my head with my feet in the air—that was the only way I could relieve the pain. It was bad. I was in sad shape."

The final blow came when George and his wife went to an auction sale where the couple bought an overstuffed chair. When George tried to pick it up, he felt something give.

It was at that point that he sought relief at any cost.

"I had developed a spinal problem, *spondylothesis*, a displacement of the spine off the sacrum," George said. "I had one of the most marked displacements in medical history: three-quarters of an inch.

"In my case, it was at least partially congenital.

"I was born with a tendency toward it, or already had it to a certain degree. But it was made worse by what I had been doing athletically.

"Whenever any doctor looked at the X-rays, they'd look at me and say, 'Be glad you're still alive and that you can even walk.'"

George's only hope was what was still considered a risky experimental procedure in 1954—a spinal fusion operation.

"Back then, the success rate was quite low," he said, "so the doctors wouldn't promise me anything except that they'd do their best. I kept postponing the operation until I couldn't put it off any longer.

"I finally had it done by Dr. Anthony J. Pisani at St. Vincent's Hospital in New York City, the orthopedic surgeon for the New York Giants. I was 38–39 years old. I was in St. Vincent's for a week and a half and was then taken by ambulance to a hospital in my hometown of Red Bank, New Jersey, about an hour away. I was there another week and a half or two weeks. They finally took me home, where I was in bed for three months.

"Finally, they said, 'Now you can take your steel brace off, go down to Florida, and sit around in the warm waters, relax, and let it mend.'"

Which is what he did. Despite the pain, George over the years had built a hugely successful mosquito-fogging operation (Fogging Unlimited, Inc.) and the equally successful Hospital Portrait Service (which eventually had more than 3,000 employees). He put trusted vice-presidents in charge of the companies and left for Fort Lauderdale.

"I'd sit in the water every day and watch the ski school on the inland waterway," George said. "Finally, the fellow who ran the school talked me into water-skiing. I was, of course, trying to beg off, saying things like, 'I'm too old. I've just had a terrible back operation.' I was feeling very sorry for myself; I was really in a state of lethargy. I was thinking I really might not ever be really viable again.

"Anyway, he did get me out and I was successful immediately because he was a good teacher with good equipment. I was just ecstatic after that. That really blew my mind, you might say. After that, I was an official advocate of water-skiing, and that's the way I have been the rest of my life. I immediately got my wife and four daughters, and took them to his ski school. He taught them all how to water-ski. Soon all six of us were skiing together behind a boat at one time. So that's the way it all started."

George continued to run his various business ventures in New Jersey, but would slip down to Florida whenever possible to water-ski. He often found himself at Cypress Gardens, a mecca for water-skiers.

"You know it is the oldest and longest-running

entertainment show in the whole world—as well as the biggest and best and grandest water-skiing show in the whole world," George said with obvious pride. "So it is a magnet for water-skiers. As a result, there are a whole bunch of water-ski schools between Orlando and Winter Haven. There's a bunch of barefoot schools, too.

"About 27–28 years ago, I came to Cypress Gardens and made maybe one guest star appearance. The next year there may have been two or three, the next year five or six, and each year I had a few more appearances. Then in 1985 I sold Hospital Portrait Service—which took pictures of babies in hospitals all over the United States and six foreign countries—and bought a small house in Florida."

The Blairs found themselves spending more and more time in Florida as George tackled water-skiing with the same enthusiasm he had lavished on earlier obsessions.

"When I was 46, I saw someone barefoot ski," he said. "Now, you understand I had been skiing about six years and had participated in a good many water-ski shows and tournaments. In fact, I had two ski schools in the New York area, in addition to my regular businesses in New Jersey. I had a number of trophies from ski competitions for regular skiing. Then I saw a guy barefooting. I thought, 'Now *that's* a real challenge.' It looked so impossible, to me, that I knew *that's* what I wanted to try.

"So I called a friend in Miami Beach who knew how to barefoot ski and asked if he'd teach me. He said, 'If you've got the will, I'll show you how.' Back then we didn't have the good suits we have now, there were no special handles, we were all just fumbling around in the dark. And at the end of the three days, they collected all my bones and put them back together again—but I knew how to barefoot!

"At once I found a whole new high and it has been one high after another. Just plain water-skiing, now that's a high for most people. And I remember the first time I could ski on one ski—that was one of my biggest highs. Then there was the first time I could stand on a dock, get pulled off on one ski—I remember that high very distinctly. But barefooting is still the highest high of all."

Today, George can barefoot for 15 minutes at a stretch.

"My feet are so tough, I'll never need a podiatrist," he told *Sports Illustrated*.

In time, "Barefootin'" George became a semi-regular—

although unpaid—performer at Cypress Gardens.

"I told them I didn't want to get paid," George said. "They said they wanted me and any time I showed up, they'd love to put me in the show. That's the arrangement we had and still have, although now for the past two or three years, they have been paying me a nominal sum.

"Some of the professional water-skiers said, 'You're a scam, you're doing these exhibitions. We get paid, but you're doing them gratis. You're just taking our money from us,' They didn't say it in so many measured words, but that's what they inferred.

"So I said to Cypress Gardens, 'Well, if you want to put me on the payroll, that's OK with me.' So they did put me on the payroll and it was lucky they did because it gives me a modicum of income, so I can at least face my wife and say I'm still a breadwinner. Since then, great things have happened to me, including my commercials for Armor All, so I hope a lot more things like that are in the wind."

In a remarkably short time, George has become one of the featured attractions at Cypress Gardens. And while he is proud of his many accomplishments at the park, one that he's most proud of is his record of durability and dependability.

"There have been so many outstanding moments, as far as pulling it off goes—I pull it off every day at Cypress Gardens," he said. "I've got a record of 98 percent perfection. They record the falls of each and every skier every day on the official record. And usually I'm at the top of that list with 98 percent successful completions."

George attributes that success ratio to his determination to always give the public the best show possible.

"I have always told my friends who were in show business or in this kind of business that they should try to do things in front of the public that they are confident they can pull off without too much trouble," he said. "So that's the way I try to operate. I try to ski within my real ability, rather than stretching my ability, in front of the crowd. There are a lot of things I do in practice when I'm training, when I'm in tournaments, or when I'm with my friends in private that I do not try to do in front of a crowd."

Not that the audiences at Cypress Gardens or the yearly eight-city Bud Water Ski Tour are ever disappointed. He opens most shows by being ripped off the beach by a speedboat going 35 miles per hour, rising to his bare feet, then circling the grandstands with the tow rope held in his teeth.

"I am considered—in my own mind, and in the minds of most of my peers in barefooting—to be the king of barefoot rope and teeth skiing because every day I do it at Cypress Gardens," George said matter-of-factly.

But it ain't braggin' if you can do it.

Although George didn't begin competing in water-ski tournaments until he was 64 years old, he now holds a host of barefoot skiing and barefoot jumping records. In 1985 he jumped 34 feet off an 18-inch ramp.

Over the years, he's broken his left ankle and eight ribs. But his worst accident came in 1987, when he broke several bones in his back. Doctors slapped him in a body cast and told him that he'd be immobilized for at least a year. Perhaps permanently.

Three months later, George was barefootin' again.

At age 77, he shows no signs of slacking up. And his list of accomplishments fills two full small-print pages. One of the highlights was his induction into the Water Ski Hall of Fame in 1991. Another was water-skiing off the coast of Antarctica. But there are many others:

"One interesting experience was skiing in the Nile with the boat operated by the two youngest sons of former president Nasser," he said. "I've skied on the Rhine River in France. I've skied the Amazon River. I've skied barefoot many times in England. And I've skied in Bombay, India, too."

In Bombay, George spun around the stinking Back Bay a few times. Then, after letting go of the tow rope, he gracefully barefoot skied to the shore.

Once there, as he told *Sports Illustrated,* a crowd of people rushed to George's side:

"Everybody wanted to touch me. It was as if they had seen Christ walking on water."

George was also the first Westerner to barefoot behind the Iron Curtain. This was in 1988, first in Bulgaria, then in the former Soviet Union, with stops on the Volga River, the Black Sea, and three different places in Moscow.

"They rolled out the red carpet for me!" George recalled. "It took a long time to get the official invitation and clearances and everything—this was before the Iron Curtain was lifted— so it wasn't easy. I dare to think this had even a minuscule influence on the raising of the Iron Curtain. I made a lot of friends there and they called me 'Mr. Banana.'

"I became an overnight celebrity, because they did a TV

show on me that was shown in 190 million homes, and that show was repeated several times. They published articles on me all over the USSR."

George's feats have also caught the attention of American television. In the past few years, he's appeared on "Live with Regis & Kathie Lee," "Stuntmasters," "Hola America" (on Univision), "CBS This Morning," "ESPN's Hot Summer Nights," "The Guinness Book of World Records," "Late Night with David Letterman," and "George Michael's Sports Machine."

"The funny part about this is, seven years ago I did a show with Arlene Francis," George said. "They sent a crew of seven, arrived at 7 a.m., spent seven hours filming me, and reduced it to seven minutes on the tube, and that show has played and played—I'll bet it has played 5,000 times. People keep calling me from all over the country saying, 'Hey, I just saw your show.' And after they describe it to me, I'll say, 'My gosh, that's 'The Time of Your Life' with Arlene Francis.

"The same thing's happened with the 'Guinness Book of World Records' show they did on me—that's been shown thousands of times all over the world, in 33 countries."

Incidentally, barefoot water-skiing may be George's primary interest, but it is not his only interest. But like barefootin', whatever George Blair does, he does in a *big* way.

"I like to iceboat in New Jersey in the wintertime," he said. "I still own two iceboats. I was the commodore and club champion of the oldest iceboat club in the world in Red Bank, which is a mecca for iceboaters. We are the oldest continuously operating iceboat club headquarters in the world for the past 120 years. All four of my daughters and all four of my grandsons enjoy the sport of iceboating and they're all good iceboaters.

"So if I'm in Florida and there is ice up there in New Jersey, if I get a chance, I'll fly up to go iceboating with them."

George attributes his seemingly inexhaustible energy to exercise and a sensible diet.

"I feel that in a way I'm a preacher, preaching the same sermon that Adele Davis does in her book, *You Are What You Eat,*" he said. "I believe that. I'm not a strict vegetarian by any stretch of the imagination, although I have one daughter who is quite strict. I eat meat once in a while, but mostly fish. I do eat what I call healthy food, that is to say unprocessed, fresh, simple, whole. And I drink an awful lot of water, more water than anybody else on the face of the earth.

"One guy once came up in San Diego and said, 'I want to

shake your hand, Mr. Blair. I'm a fireman, and we've been watching your Armor All commercial. All of those guys down there watch you operate at 77 and they're going to stop drinking so much and get some healthy habits going.'

"Maybe they'll pass the word on to their children."

There is one other small, insignificant component to George's diet. The banana. George Blair is *consumed* by bananas. Or is it the other way around?

"As a result of the fact that bananas are yellow and that they are God's most nearly perfect food, I have an affinity for bananas, too," he said. "They're very easy to carry, the package is biodegradable, so it was natural for me to gravitate to bananas. They are 75 percent water. You can grab one while you're out there water-skiing or barefooting. It's like having a water jug with you on a hot day. It gives you water and energy from the sucrose. It also gives you potassium for your muscles.

"As a result of my affinity for yellow and bananas, I give away about two tons of bananas each year. In September 1990, Chiquita called me and said, 'We've been reading about you and seeing you on the tube. What is this thing you have about bananas?'

"I said, 'Do you know how long I've been waiting for this call? About 27 years.'

"They said, 'What can we do for you?'

"I said, 'You can start by furnishing my bananas.'

"They said, 'Well, how many?'

"And I said, 'Oh, about two tons a year.'

"They said, 'Where do you want them sent?'

"I said, 'I'll let you know.' And I have."

So wherever George goes, whether it is to perform or to compete in a water-skiing tournament, he calls up Chiquita and they send him bananas. *Lots* of bananas.

There has been some talk about George doing commercials for Chiquita, but that hasn't materialized yet.

George says that it is getting close to time to prepare for the second show at Cypress Gardens, but he has a few parting words of wisdom:

"My advice to young people is to have a focus, set goals, and do it," he said.

"My advice to 60-year-olds who want to be doing this is, 'There is hope for all of us, even me.' Every day I try to do a little better. And you ought to, too. Start easy, but go for it. And set goals.

"I still have all kinds of goals. I can't wait to test myself with the next goal, with the next accomplishment. I've got all kinds of things I want to be doing. There are not enough seconds in each minute, not enough minutes in each hour, for me to do what I want to do. That's my problem."

That, and how to get rid of two tons of free bananas each year.

Chapter 5

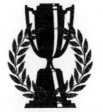

Sister Madonna Buder

SPOKANE, WASHINGTON—Sister Madonna Buder was well on her way to another record in the women's 60–64 age bracket in her latest Ironman. Sister Madonna "visualizes" her finishing times and has been remarkably close on a number of occasions.

She was well ahead of that pace when she came upon a distraught, dehydrated competitor by the side of the track. She stopped, comforted the woman, and stayed with her until medical attention arrived. Then Sister Madonna continued her run.

In the end, she *still* broke the Ironman record for her age bracket, though she missed her envisioned predicted time by about as long as it took her to render aid.

This is the remarkable story of Sister Madonna, 62, the top woman's Ironman athlete of recent years. It's not your usual biography. But then, she's not your usual Catholic nun, either. And she may be the only Ironman competitor for whom competing isn't an obsession. It is, instead, a form of living prayer.

Sister Madonna Buder was born Dorothy Marie Buder, only daughter of Gustavus and Kathryn Marie Buder, two pillars of old St. Louis society. As Dorothy, Sister Madonna was born to ride horses and won numerous awards for her riding and showmanship.

"I just was always an active individual," she said. "My father, I suppose, bred it into me because he was a champion oarsman. And that's supposed to be one of the toughest sports of all. My mother was an oarsman's widow, so to speak, until the boathouse burned down.

"And it came naturally to me to be active, to enjoy the outdoors. My mother still enjoys nature a whole lot. My mother was drawn to my father because he used to take her on interesting trips while they were dating."

After teaching one year of first grade and fending off a marriage proposal or two, Sister Madonna joined the Sisters of the Good Shepherd at age 23. The Good Shepherd nuns are a semi-cloistered order dedicated to helping young girls in need. Sister Madonna celebrated her Silver Jubilee with the order in 1981. In 1986, she transferred to the Sisters for Christian Community.

"With the Sisters for Christian Community, which was established in 1970," she said, "I find that our gift is to melt in with the rest of the populace right in the marketplace. I figure that's just what I'm doing, mixing in with these triathletes."

Even during her days with the Sisters of the Good Shepherd, Sister Madonna remained fitness-conscious. But she didn't begin running seriously until 1978, at age 48.

"I was introduced to running through a Catholic priest who was attending a pyscho-dynamics workshop on the Oregon coast where the Sisters had a beach house," she said. "He had come in from running and was expounding on the benefits of running, but he was talking as if it were a panacea for everything that ails you.

"I said, 'Wait a minute! I've been active all my life—but I enjoy interactive sports. I can't see getting up there and running for no good reason.'"

But the priest challenged her to try it—and she did, running apparently effortlessly along the beach for half a mile.

Sister Madonna continued running after that, gradually working up to four miles a day in hand-me-down tennis shoes.

"One day when I came back from working in a photo lab where I was doing my own processing, I saw a poster advertising the second Bloomsday Run here in Spokane—I hadn't even known there was a first!" she said. "It pictured all these people running elbow to elbow and it just repulsed me. I thought, 'My gosh, it's hard enough to run without having to elbow your way through a mass like that!'

"But the more I rejected it, the more it clung to me. Then I got a long-distance phone call from my mother who was alerting me to the fact that the marriage of one of my brothers was in jeopardy. I told her, 'It really doesn't surprise me, I've seen it coming for about five years.' I attributed it to an unacknowledged alcoholism problem.

"Suddenly, I said, 'I think I'm going to run this run here in Spokane as the living Way of the Cross, hoping that the Lord will take my will to endure and transfer it to my brother, that he will have the will to give up his dependency on alcohol. My mother said, 'Honey, how far is this?' I said, 'Mom, it's 8.2 miles.' She said, 'You can't do that.' I said, 'I won't know until I try.'"

Sister Madonna's unexpected promise came only five weeks after she began running, but it sustained her through the difficult days ahead.

"All of the training I was doing was in cheap, non-shock tennis shoes," she said. "By week four, my knees were so large I couldn't bend them back and my calves so tight I couldn't even indent them.

"One week later, I was laid out on the floor attempting to do yoga exercises—which I had been doing all along, without realizing this was like engaging in warmups—when I just couldn't push my body to do another thing at that point. So I just collapsed in tears. I said, 'Lord, I can't! I can't! My whole body is rebelling.'"

In the privacy of her room, Sister Madonna continued to pour her heart out in prayer. Suddenly, a still, small voice cut through her tears.

"The voice said, 'In My agony in the garden, I did not know how many people down through the ages would respond to My act of love. I had to step out in faith—even as you do.'

"I said, 'All right, Lord, You win. But You've got to be my strength because I can't do it.'

"It took all I had to wrench myself from the bed, go downstairs and set my feet outside the side door. After this struggle, I eventually came back feeling no worse than when I had left. How could I?"

Just before the Bloomsday Run, a friend of the order took Sister Madonna shopping for a better pair of shoes. The only ones that fit were a $12 pair of house-brand tennis shoes. She tried to break them in before the race.

"With just a few days left to Bloomsday, besides my enlarged knees and tight calves, I now had blisters to contend with," she said. "But the day of the race was more like the Resurrection than the Passion of our Lord. The weather was about 70 degrees, with a bright, cloudless sky. So I got through the race—and not too badly—especially for someone who periodically walked for several minutes every two miles. But the camaraderie of the race was just really fun.

"At the end of the race the organizers were passing out

entry forms for other races. I thought, 'I don't ever want to put myself through this agony again.'

"But then I thought, 'I've already got these crazy-looking tennis shoes, so I might as well get some use out of them.' I'll just enter one race a month! And that's how it all started."

As with many runners, one race a month eventually became two races a month. And two became three. And more.

"Then I had a ridiculous thought: 'I wonder if I could do a marathon by the time I reach 50?'" she asked herself. Quite sensibly, she set her sights on the best-known marathon in the world—the Boston Marathon.

In 1981, women aged 40 and over had to qualify for Boston by running a sub 3 hour and 30 minute marathon. Sister Madonna's first marathon was a year later in Coeur d'Alene, Idaho. Two years later, she qualified for Boston with 46 seconds to spare. She entered and ran in both the 1982 and '83 Marathons.

"I completed my first Boston Marathon and, at age 52, was probably the first Catholic nun to do so—but it wasn't easy," she said. "It didn't start until noon and the only things I had had to eat were a banana, some milk, and a granola bar at about 6 a.m. Before the race even started, I was conscious of being hungry while crunched up in the crowd!

"By the time I hit mile 24, I was probably consuming my own body fat. At this point my legs turned to absolute lead. I've learned a lot since then. Those last two miles were absolute torture. I still did it in a respectable 3 hours and 31 minutes— which included the extra six minutes it took to get to the starting line after the gun went off. Not bad for my age group, but those last two miles certainly put me in touch with the Lord's willingness to carry the cross to Calvary for our sakes!"

When she returned home, she noticed an article in the newspaper about an upcoming "troika"—a 1.2-mile swim, a 56-mile bike ride, and a 13.1-mile run.

"I thought that I had done the epitome of foolishness by engaging in a marathon, but this took the cake as far as the height of physical extravagance goes," Sister Madonna said with a laugh. "However, upon further reflection, I figured, 'Heck, I've done these marathons, I used to swim and use my mother's balloon-tire bike as a child, so why not try it?'

"So I borrowed one of the oversize bikes that the girls never used, not realizing that not having a frame to fit my frame wasn't the smartest thing to do. Breaking myself into using a

10-speed bike was like breaking in a colt. The difference between the bikes I was used to and a 10-speed was like going from a pony to a racehorse. And I've been learning about 10-, 12-, 14-, 18-speed bikes—there is no end to it as the technology improves. But that's what got me started."

Serious bicycling, however, involves some risk. Sister Madonna has endured five major bike accidents and crashes. The most recent was October 29, 1992, shortly after returning from another Ironman, where she set a new age-group record of 13 hours, 19 minutes, and one second.

"This accident was caused by a huge dog leaping across my path, which I couldn't possibly avoid," she said. "If it had not been for my helmet, which took the brunt of the crash and split open, I wouldn't be here to tell the tale."

Her first serious bike accident prevented her from competing in the 1984 Ironman. Her goal had been to dedicate each leg of the triathlon for a different benefit: the heart, lung, and diabetes associations.

"On June 1984, I suffered a broken scapula, a broken jaw, a compound-fractured elbow, and multiple abrasions and bruises while training on a borrowed bike back in St. Louis while visiting my parents for their 55th wedding anniversary," Sister Madonna said. "So now I simply dedicate each leg of the triathlon to one of my three brothers by way of a continuous prayer for them, hoping in this way, that I might alleviate some of the problems in their lives.

"When I had my second bike accident, I didn't know if I'd ever be able to walk again. The doctors never really gave me the go-ahead signal to engage in these activities again—I just went and did it. When it comes to training on the bike, you can't really get into it heavy without your number coming up sooner or later."

Strangely enough, Sister Madonna's bad luck seems to run in seven-year cycles.

"My first three bad accidents followed close on one another in 1984," she said. "I'd just recover from one shock when the next would occur. That included the death of my father in the same time frame. As a consequence of those accidents, it took four years before my broken hip was used to all of the 'scrap metal' surrounding it. I hope I'll never have to repeat another 1984–85 again. I think I've done enough penance for the rest of my life!

"But in 1991, He almost took my mother home around the

same date that He took my father, which was seven years earlier. I had another bike crash that upset me late in the 1991 season, then this one in October 1992. I certainly hope a third accident isn't lurking ahead somewhere in this seven-year cycle. I find myself crying out to the Lord, 'When is enough, enough?'"

Fortunately, she's found sympathetic doctors who not only bind her wounds, but encourage her participation in triathlons.

"Actually, two of the doctors who have eased me through my traumas here in Spokane are triathlete competitors themselves!" she said. "I've managed to beat both of them in competition—and they're just young sprites! They encourage my activities.

"The doctor who was responsible for tending my compound-fractured elbow in St. Louis, however, cautioned me not to rush into things. Three weeks later I was entered in the Diet Pepsi Championships in New York, so I put my arm in a sling and a sign on my back that said, 'Beware, injured runner! No passing on right, please!' And I tried to run as far to the right as I could. Only a handful of people passed me on the right during the whole 10K, and I came in fourth due to the extra precautions. I never told my doctor."

Through August 1992, Sister Madonna had completed 13 Ironman competitions, including three in Hawaii, along with 29 separate marathons.

"Someday, now that I know I can do the Hawaiian Ironman well, I would like to break the 13-hour barrier," she said. "I figure if I don't give in to myself in the marathon portion, I should be able to do it.

"That will be my goal for my next Ironman, whether it is in Canada, Hawaii, or New Zealand. Right now, I'm just lucky to be alive!

Sister Madonna's story is unusual in yet another way. Unlike so many other marathon and triathlon athletes, she doesn't have a formal exercise schedule. Instead, her *life* is her exercise schedule.

"I compete in one Ironman triathlon after another during the season, so I use one to train for the next one," she said. "During the rest of the year, I use my legs and wheels to literally run errands, to church, to the post office. Of course, if the groceries are too heavy, I have to take a car. Otherwise, though, anything I can do either by running or biking, I do. It is not unusual for me to do a mini-triathlon as I go about my day, especially if it is one of the three or four days each week I also go swimming.

"I figure this keeps me on maintenance until the season starts up again. When you get to my age, you don't have to go out and do hard-core training like the younger set. If I'm just consistent, this keeps the body less susceptible to fatigue and injuries—unless I encounter the unforeseen! And I'm getting a little tired of encountering the asphalt!"

Her diet is equally unstructured.

"I don't actually have a strict diet regimen, but I eat simply," Sister Madonna said. "I mostly eat carbohydrates, fresh vegetables—I grow my own in season—and fresh fruits. I do have a weakness that sets in in the colder weather, however. I will sometimes give in to chocolate candies, chocolate chip cookies, and ice cream—although I've switched to frozen yogurt.

"I will eat meat if I am out with friends, but I only cook it sparingly myself, maybe twice a week. I just try to keep a well-rounded diet, but I do believe in vitamin supplements."

The only downside to Sister Madonna's remarkable feats of fitness and health—and she could pass for 20 years younger—is that there have been very few women competing in the triathlons in her age bracket.

"Sometimes I end up mostly competing with myself in the age groups I've been in," she said. "I was very happy to see my age group begin to grow. I certainly welcome this increase. I don't like to be up on the podium all by myself! It thrills me to see others join the ranks. During the 1991 senior sports championships, there was actually a field of 11 in my age group for that triathlon sprint!"

Shortly after this interview was completed, Sister Madonna (who was born July 24, 1930), wrote me an excited note, saying that a 69-year-old, Lynn Edwards, had completed the 1992 Hawaiian Ironman—the first woman that age to do so.

When she's not swimming across lagoons or running over mountains, Sister Madonna stays active in her order as a pastoral counselor, with both a media ministry and a prison ministry as part of the Omega Outreach Program.

As a result, she often finds herself speaking with young people, some of whom express an interest in her extraordinary fitness level.

"I tell them, 'Get out and do it! You'll never regret it! What's keeping you from it? Start now. It's never too late to start—

never!' Some of the most inspirational people are these older ones who didn't start until they were 50–60 years old. There were 11 triathletes entered in the 70-plus bracket for men for the '92 Hawaiian Ironman and all but three finished. Amazing!

"My concern is that the young ones, the pros—if they keep pushing themselves like they are, by the time they reach my age they will be burned out, unless they ease back and start up again later in life. It is fun to get better with each succeeding year."

Not surprisingly, that's much the same advice she gives to people nearing retirement age.

"I say, 'Go for it! Just listen to your body, it will tell you what to do and how far you can take it. Be patient and it will respond to your commands, but don't bite off more than you can chew. Begin gradually and each day, each week, set a little goal for yourself and then increase the margin. Your body does need to get acquainted with that kind of anaerobic and aerobic exercise you are introducing to it. Once you get synchronized, there is no end to what you can do.

"Just be reasonable in your expectations. What might be good for one might not be good for another. We're all individuals. Do respect yourself as such."

But to succeed in changing your life for the better, Sister Madonna maintains that there needs to be a serious motivation underlying that change. She says there needs to be as much mental discipline as physical discipline.

"Whatever your intention is for beginning this exercise regime, you do need to have some intentions or goals," she said.

"For myself, it happened to a spiritual intention that got me started. It is my belief that you can spiritualize anything you do, depending on the intention with which you do it. I contend that when you discover you have a certain gift or talent or skill, you owe it to your Creator to perfect it as much as possible to give honor and glory to the Supreme Gift-Giver.

"It has been a real discovery and growth process for me, all of these struggles, to reach the peak where I am now. I have come to realize in a more realistic way what Jesus endured for our sakes, what He went through to redeem us."

But for Sister Madonna, "spiritualizing" her triathlons doesn't mean competing in a traditional nun's habit.

"Well, I'm not nearly as squeamish about wearing close-fitting tights as I used to be, because they have become so common these days," she said. "Rather than stand out in a crowd, I prefer to blend in with the rest of the scenery and wear what the rest of the triathletes wear—barring bikinis, of course. If you're going to do what the others do, you dress as they dress."

Still, Sister Madonna *can't* help it. Somehow, she *does* stand out in the crowds of runners and triathletes. Her gentle nature, her affirming words, her positive, supportive attitude often draw other competitors to her. In the end, her running has become yet another form of ministry.

"It has provided me occasions to minister to others, but I didn't consciously go out intending it would be that way," she said. "It just happened spontaneously. Twice during marathons, knowing that I am a religious person, people have started to bare their souls to me. Sometimes talking helps take their minds off the painful accumulation of mileage, as running helps relieve them of their personal problems—at least temporarily. I just happen to be out in the marketplace with them and accessible to their needs.

"In two different Ironman events, I've stopped to help a struggling competitor until adequate help was available. But it is a two-way street, and I've also been a recipient of others' compassion.

"It keeps me in touch with the beauty and the beast in our human makeup. The drama of these events reveals the bare bones of our nature, alternating between pain and exhilaration. And I continue to enjoy the nuances of life to the fullest."

Not that she's any plastic saint, of course. Sister Madonna knows the pains and petty grievances of day-to-day life, just like the rest of us. And, when the weather changes, the screws, and plates and bolts in her elbow remind her once again, as if she ever forgot, about her own, all-too-frail, humanity.

"When they exhume me for canonization, they'll know who they've got," she cheerily told the *St. Louis Post–Dispatch*.

Chapter 6

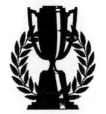

Hulda Crooks

LOMA LINDA, CALIFORNIA—Two mountains claim Hulda Crooks. The elfin 96-year-old is affectionately known as "Grandma Whitney" in the United States and "Grandma Fuji" in Japan.

And Hulda Crooks claims at least one of those mountains herself. In 1991, Congress officially designated one of Mt. Whitney's peaks as Crooks Peak. In doing so, the government broke with long-standing tradition against naming geographic formations after a still-living person.

But if anyone has earned that honor, it is Hulda. At age 91, she climbed Mt. Whitney's 14,494 feet for the 23rd time—only six weeks after climbing Japan's Mt. Fuji.

Today, her mountain-climbing days are behind her. But Hulda Crooks continues to astound her fellow residents in her Loma Linda nursing home with her prodigious daily walks, keen, penetrating mind, and deep, abiding religious faith.

It wasn't always this way. For much of her life, Hulda was shy and introspective, self-conscious about her weight, a bookworm who happily remained in the background. Most of the dramatic changes happened late in her life.

Hulda's German-born parents fled Russia and made their way to Canada's still sparsely settled western provinces in the 1880s.

"My father said it was time to get out from under the paw of the Russian bear," she recalled. "So they made their way to Saskatchewan, Canada, to begin their life over in a new—and free—country. I was born May 19, 1896, in Saskatchewan. My father was a farmer. I worked on the farm growing up."

Her father later opened a country store, allowing young Hulda free access to the hard-candy barrel and chocolate box, as well as the rich cream, butter, milk, and eggs that are part and parcel of the self-sustaining farm. When the five-foot Hulda moved away at age 18, she weighed a robust 160 pounds.

"When I left home, I had only completed five grades of country schooling," she said. "I had to get my schooling after I left home because my father didn't have a formal education in Russia—he had virtually none at all. He was self-educated, but he could beat most any lawyer in an argument. He learned to speak five languages: his natural German, Russian, Ukranian, Polish, and English. I grew up speaking German; I didn't know English until I was around 10.

"Since my father didn't have a formal education and he had to do it on his own, he wasn't much concerned about his children's education. They could do it the way he did: on their own! His idea of the education a girl needed was to learn to read and write and do a little figuring and make a good soup for her husband! And that was it!

"My father had taken me out of school when I was able to read and write and figure—as he thought that was enough—so that I could work at his country store. He put me in as a clerk because I could figure the price of things and keep track of things we sold on credit to the Ukranian people who lived all around us. They would pay it back in the fall when they harvested their crops. That's all the education my father thought was necessary for me."

Hulda and her brother Ed had been raised as Lutherans, but a Seventh-Day Adventist Bible study convinced them to leave their father's denomination.

"When my father found out that we were interested in the Seventh-Day Adventist teaching, he said: 'Quit going to those meetings. Or go—and don't come back!' So that's what Ed and I did. And it was the last time I lived at home. I wasn't quite 18. After that, we had to get our own education.

"If you know anything about Seventh-Day Adventists, you know they are strong on education. So immediately Ed and I were inspired to get an education. We had no financial backing and did it on our own."

The two eventually made their way to the United States. After a year at Pacific Union College in California, Hulda transferred to Loma Linda University (near Riverside, California). She chose the school because it was the only Adventist college offering classes in dietary science or dietetics.

"It took me three years to do two years' worth of school because I had to work to pay bills," Hulda said. "I got sick. I got pneumonia and lost nearly a whole year of schooling at

Loma Linda. But I went back to it and I eventually completed a Bachelor of Science in dietetics in 1927. My brother Eddie eventually became a medical doctor."

Hulda was soon attracted to the work of Dr. Mervyn G. Hardinge of the School of Health at Loma Linda University and went to work for him in his lab. Dr. Hardinge would publish nearly 40 major articles—generally on nutrition—and present 15 papers at professional conferences through the 1970s. Hulda collaborated on eight of them, including several important early studies on both fiber and fat in the diet.

Coupled with her strict Adventist teachings, Hulda's research with Dr. Hardinge convinced her to stand firm in her decision to become a lacto-ovo-vegetarian.

"I haven't had a mouthful of meat, fish, or fowl since before I was 18," she said. "The animals get their food from vegetarian sources and when we eat meat, we get it second-hand! And so we vegetarians have learned to make many interesting dishes that are the main dish, the protein dish. We eat all kinds of different things. Of course, you don't need to. You could eat very simply. I use milk. Maybe a cup a day. There are protein dishes from beans, peas, and greens. If you're not a vegetarian, you'd be surprised what tasty dishes vegetarians make out of the plant foods."

Along the way, Hulda married Samuel A. Crooks, then a recent graduate of medical school. Samuel was plagued with a coronary condition that limited his activity, yet he urged Hulda to spend time outdoors. He also awakened her interest in the flora and fauna of the region. In time, she could identify every flower, every bird in Southern California. The couple were married for 23 years before his sudden death in 1950.

"I started climbing mountains because of my husband," she said. He pushed me out to do things on my own. He couldn't go climb mountains with me because of his heart problems, but he pushed me to do it. And so I began climbing our local mountain—the highest in Southern California, called San Gorgonio (elevation 11,845 feet)—and I've climbed that at least 30 times over the years. I enjoyed it immediately. It wasn't hard for me, I didn't get too tired, and I enjoyed it."

As Hulda told *Life and Health* Magazine, her late-blooming interest in mountain-climbing helped her cope with the loss of her beloved husband: "Alone, I carried on as best I could and as I knew he had expected me to. My familiarity with nature and my love for the outdoors helped tranquilize my emotions."

The mountains' calming, uplifting effects were not lost on Hulda's friends. Soon she found herself invited on serious hiking expeditions on a regular basis.

Her health, once tenuous, continued to improve. Her weight melted away. And, once she discovered that she felt best when she walked regularly, she sold her car.

The mountain that held the most attraction for her was Mt. Whitney, the highest peak in the contiguous 48 states. Her interest was originally piqued by an offhand comment her late husband had made years earlier. Her daily walks on the Loma Linda campus only intensified her desire to climb Whitney.

"Now and then I heard (the students) talk of climbing Mt. Whitney and I wondered whether maybe I could do it too," Hulda later told *Life and Health*. "But the years slipped by and with them the likelihood of my ever trying."

Her chance finally came in an unexpected invitation from two old friends, Carolyn Stuyvesant and Gerry Lohrke. The year was 1962. Hulda was 66.

"I had heard the medical students and the nurses talking about climbing Mt. Whitney, but I was always afraid to ask to go because I was afraid I'd be a nuisance on the trail, that I couldn't do it," she said. "And so I had never asked to go. But when these two lady acquaintances and climbers asked me to go with them, I thought that it was safe for me to try it. I made it. And that got me hooked on it."

Hulda eventually climbed Mt. Whitney 23 times, the last time at age 91, six weeks after she'd climbed Mt. Fuji in Japan. She climbed Mt. Whitney every year from 1962 to 1982, save for 1965. In 1968 she climbed it twice, including one climb with brothers Ed (75) and Chris (77)!

In time, Hulda began adding other approaches to Whitney and other ranges to her already impressive list of climbs. In 1971, at age 75, she crossed the range over Kearsarge Pass (11,800 feet) and down to the John Muir Trail. She then followed the Trail to Forester Pass (13,200 feet), down to Crab Tree and up Mt. Whitney. Total distance: 55 miles.

A year later she crossed the Great Western Divide, went down the Kern River, up to the top of Whitney, and down to the Portal, a distance of 80 miles, carrying a full backpack.

At age 86 (1982), Hulda hiked 40 miles over Cottonwood Pass (11,211 feet), down Crab Tree, up the Muir Trail, and back up to the top of Whitney again.

The 23 Whitney trips included early snowstorms, late thunderstorms, trails damaged by earthquakes and rock slides, and an increasing amount of media coverage. NBC filmed her 1979 climb all of the way to the summit. Footage from her trek aired on both the evening and morning news programs. It was followed by an appearance on "The Tonight Show with Johnny Carson."

The 1981 trip was also filmed and included a "Good Morning, America" greeting from the summit for that popular morning show.

From ages 81 to 91, she also climbed 90 of the highest peaks in Southern California as part of a small, select group of hikers who vowed to climb all 268 Southern California peaks and high points between the elevations of 5,000 and 11,500-plus feet.

Hulda has also participated in a number of half and quarter marathons and road races.

In 1987, at age 91, Hulda climbed Mt. Fuji. The ascent was sponsored by Densu, Inc., Japan's largest advertising company.

"Hundreds of Densu employees had been climbing Mt. Fuji, Japan's sacred mountain, every year," Hulda recalled. "They had been climbing it every year for 60 years and the company wanted to celebrate their 60th anniversary, but they hadn't decided *how* to celebrate it.

"The Densu people were also interested in vegetarianism and I've been a vegetarian since I was 18. They were also interested in Adventism—and I was an Adventist!

"It was the most unusual climb I ever took. Densu is an advertising company, so they made sure the world knew about it—they really publicized it. The world was watching this climb! It was fun."

The small party climbing Fuji included an Adventist doctor from Tokyo. Advertising agency or not, Hulda suspected that it wouldn't be good publicity to have a 91-year-old climber hurt while in Densu's care!

"The first day was our longest one," she said. "The next day we stopped short of the summit because we wanted to be there for the sunrise. The climb took two days and a little bit of a third day. We came down the same day that we watched the sunrise.

"Many people recognize me now when they see me after all of that. But if they don't, and someone introduces me as the woman who climbed Mt. Fuji, they know that immediately."

When she had climbed Mt. Whitney earlier that year, she believed it would be the final time. But in August 1991, she was flown by U.S. Army Chinook helicopter to a trail camp about 2,000 feet below the Whitney peak. Once there, she was met by a large and vocal party of friends and dignitaries for the formal naming of Crooks Peak.

"It's been a great inspiration for me," she told a *Los Angeles Times* reporter later that day. "When I come down from the mountain, I feel like I can battle in the valley again."

And later still, as she looked wistfully back at Whitney from the tiny town of Lone Pine, she whispered to the reporter: "There's *my* mountain."

And it is.

Today at 96, Hulda Crooks has decided her mountain-climbing days are over. But not her life.

"I still climb 16 stair steps to the second floor of my retirement villa many times a day instead of riding on the elevator," she says proudly. "I leave the elevator for the *old* folks. Not many of them are as old as I am, of course!

"I walk each day. I can walk, I suppose, about two miles. I think I could walk more if I had to. I don't think that I would want to. I walk over to the veterans' hospital near Loma Linda. There are ponds on both sides of the hospital and there are ducks and swans and different things that are of interest to me. That's where I usually walk every morning. I go clear around the Veteran's Hospital."

On other days, she may walk further still.

"I walk to the Loma Linda Market, which is probably three-quarters of a mile, so it is a mile and a half walk round trip," Hulda said. "Most of the folks here who are much younger than I am would take the van there from the retirement home.

"We have about a hundred people here. Two or three times a week the van takes them to the track to walk. But I don't go with them because there's nothing to see. You just go round and round and round! So I go on my own to the veterans' hospital where I can see more interesting things."

In recent days at the ponds, Hulda has seen two blue herons, a pair of black swans, some white swans, and a pair of female wood ducks. And she knows all of the flowers she sees along the way by name, too.

Not surprisingly, Hulda's prodigious feats have drawn the attention of doctors as well as reporters. A VO_2 max test (VO_2

max is a measurement of a body's ability to use oxygen during exercise) conducted on her at age 90 revealed a reading close to that of the average 60-year-old woman.

"My doctor is an Adventist," she said. "I don't know, but I imagine he's a vegetarian too. I think about 50 percent of Seventh Day Adventists are. He is supportive of what I've done. My doctor, Roy Jutzy, has been my doctor for many, many years. He's really a heart specialist.

"I will say that I have a little heart problem. Dr. Jutzy told me, the last time I saw him, that if I were young, he would do surgery. There is something—and I don't know what it is—that evidently I was born with, the narrowing of something that makes it harder for the heart to bounce the blood around. Certainly, that hasn't amounted to much over 96 years! So I can't complain with all of the mountains I've climbed and all of the walking that I've done. I've hiked many, many miles (and) it hasn't given me much trouble."

Hulda's legions of friends and family members have been very supportive.

She says, incidentally, that she prefers walking and hiking with people closer to her own age.

"Of course, a lot of them don't do much hiking now," she said, "so I go mostly by myself. Mostly because younger people either want to go faster than I can go, or they want to go slower, or they're not interested in what I want to see."

Ultimately, any conversation with Hulda Crooks returns to the center point of her life.

"My religious faith is very, very important to me," she said, "in all of my decisions in life. It *is* my life. I don't know what I would do without it. I would have no outlet. I'm now nearing the end of my life at 96. If I had no hope for the future, what would I do?

"I dedicated my life to the Lord when I was young. And all these years through life's problems and disappointments, this has steadied me and upheld me. I don't know where I would have gone if it hadn't been for that faith."

The Bible, Hulda believes, teaches that our bodies are the temple of the Holy Ghost. That's one reason she's maintained her marvelous level of physical fitness.

"And your body can deteriorate like a temple can deteriorate if you let it get full of trash and whatnot," she said. "You have people putting a lot of trash into their bodies: smoking, drinking, and eating foods that are not good. They don't take very good care of their temples. But the Lord expects us to. If we ruin them, we deprive the Lord of the service we might give to others and to Him.

"If I should come up with fatal cancer now, it wouldn't shake my faith. The Lord is the boss of my body. I've tried to live healthily. From the time that I surrendered my life to the Lord when I was not quite 18, I've never questioned that. I have never given that up; I have never taken back that surrender."

"You know, the Bible says the Lord's righteousness is like the great mountains," she told the *Los Angeles Times* after the ceremony at Mt. Whitney. "There is no limit to it. I give credit to my faith in the Lord that I've been able to survive so many years. What credit people try to give to me, I turn right over to the Lord."

She can try to deflect it, of course, but some credit will always reflect back on the little lady from Loma Linda with a heart the size of Mt. Whitney.

Chapter 7

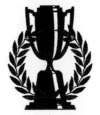

Norton Davey

OCEAN HILLS, CALIFORNIA—At 74, F. Norton Davey is one of the world's premier Ironman triathletes. In addition to winning a number of triathlons, he's also a world-class marathoner in his age group. He is blessed—or cursed—with a burning desire not just to compete, but to win.

Just how "burning" is that desire? Consider this story from 1987 when Norton was 69 years old:

"I have for many years been active in hiking and mountain climbing and trekking of a non-technical nature," he recalled. "Some years ago I got rather serious about it because I enjoyed it so, and I wanted to do a little more of it. So I went over to Africa and tried to climb Mount Kilimanjaro. I flunked it. I got to within 600 feet of the top and couldn't make the summit, which is about 19,300 feet.

"So, a year and a half later, I tried a different route and I couldn't make that, either. So I came back down to the bottom, and the group I had come with was returning home and I was so disappointed, almost crushed, that they had made it and I had not. Of course, there was the fact that I was about 30 years older than any of the rest of them!

"At the last minute, I canceled my return flight reservations, which were hard to get over there in the best of times, went back to the base of the mountain, hired another guide and two porters, and went up to the top! I like to think of that as one of my more persevering achievements, physically."

But then, that's the sort of story you'd expect from a 74-year-old who annually runs what many consider the most grueling marathon in the world—the Catalina Marathon—just for fun!

Norton was born in New Rochelle, New York, but grew up

in Plainfield, New Jersey, in a family with four children. His father was an insurance executive in New York City. Norton was active in gymnastics and calisthenics at the local YMCA in Plainfield through the Junior Leaders Club.

"It was sponsored by a very active physician in Plainfield who did a great deal for many of us who were tall, skinny kids who would get broken apart on a football field!" Norton said.

After high school, he attended Syracuse University in upstate New York.

"I was reasonably active in college," Norton said. "I did row on the varsity crew at Syracuse. I again tried out for football, but I was too skinny to take that constant physical abuse. So I got my exercise and did quite well by sitting down and rowing backwards!

"I also made an early profession change: I was pre-med at Syracuse and had one year at med school before I realized that medical school and I did not go together. I realized that medicine was not for me so I got out. Just about that time the war came along and that temporarily shelved my career decisions!"

Norton eventually flew airplanes through two wars, and actually maintained flying status until 1989. At various times along the way, he's flown light airplanes, from the tip of Mexico to Alaska, and from Nova Scotia to Los Angeles.

But before he went off to World War II, Norton married another Plainfield native, Betty.

"After the war, Betty and I started driving west from New Jersey one day and we stopped in Denver for 15 years," he said. "There three of our four children were born.

"And there we developed a love for the Colorado mountains. As a result, we spent a lot of time hiking. We aren't technical climbers, we just enjoy the outside. We fished and hiked and spent two or three, sometimes four weekends per month up in the mountains during the summer season. We were a very close-knit family and we had a great time with that."

Fortunately, mountain climbing wasn't all that Norton did while in Colorado. He also received a master's degree in accounting at the University of Denver and worked as an accountant until retiring in 1982.

Eventually, the hiking gave way to snow skiing. But as he got older, Norton found that the physical demands of skiing were interfering with his enjoyment of the sport. As a last resort, he considered taking up running to build up his legs.

"The running really started when my company's medical director—I was with Continental Airlines at that time and had been for 20 years—suggested I get some exercise because of some unusual chest feelings I had and also because of some EKG results," Norton said.

"I said, 'Exercise? I haven't got time for exercise!' I was working 80 hours a week at a desk and was traveling just about all over the world. But the doctor said, 'No, you've got to do something. Have you tried running?' I looked at him and I said, 'Hey, you're a physician and with all of your credentials, you're saying a crazy thing like telling a 55-year-old to start running?'"

Norton doesn't remember the doctor's exact words, but they included an emphatic Yes!

"So I did and I discovered three things: First, it was good for me. It brought down my weight, my blood pressure, and it relieved a lot of tension I had with business. The second thing I found was that I was actually enjoying it. And then, about two or three years after I started, the worst thing of all happened—I got competitive! I ran my first race and from there on it was, 'Look out! Here I come!'"

It wasn't long before Norton's running habit grew into a full-fledged addiction. In 1978 came the final stage for anyone with a running dependency—the marathon.

"I ran my first marathon in early '78 and enjoyed it so much that I did eight or nine more during the rest of that year!" he said. "I didn't know any better, and as a result, it didn't help my physical condition any. I was plagued with colds and I finally went back to my medical director who said, 'Take it easy; you're overdoing it. You go from nothing to everything!'

"We cut it back to three or four marathons a year. So, through mid-1992, I've run 50–55 marathons."

Those 50–55 marathons have featured the full gamut of outcomes. He's had exceptional times and horrible times. He's run in idyllic conditions and hideous conditions. One February marathon in Seaside, Oregon, nearly ended in tragedy. About halfway through the race in the chilling weather, Norton began suffering from hypothermia. Fortunately, Betty realized that something was wrong, hunted him down in their car, and warmed him up before any damage was done.

"The one great success I've had will always remain in my memory," he said. "Like most marathoners who have not run the Boston Marathon, to do that becomes a goal. Simply to run in the Boston and to finish—because the Boston is the granddaddy of them all, and it has been around over 100 years—is a dream.

"But the Boston Marathon, because of the running craze that was coming along about then, was very difficult to enter. I applied and was refused. I was told that I had to have a certain time for my age at some other marathon in order to qualify for the Boston. That time happened to be 3 hours and 30 minutes. I had never run anything under 3:40, so it just seemed out of the question—unless I went in as what they called a 'Boston Bandit.'"

In desperation, with the cut-off date for the Boston Marathon looming, Norton applied for the New York Marathon.

"I got lucky that day," he said. "I remember it well. In fact, if you've got time, I'll tell you about every step along the way! But I ran the 26 miles in 3:27, so I made my cut-off by three minutes and that was my entry into Boston. Running in Boston wasn't nearly as much of an accomplishment as was qualifying for Boston! I think most people will tell you the same thing: Boston was just something to do after that!

"But I got there and I had another great day at the Boston Marathon. I ran a 3:35, and while numbers don't mean a lot, it was fun to be there. That was my one attempt at Boston. I've thought about going back, 12 years later, but we'll see."

In 1981, Norton was plagued with a slight running injury that kept him off the streets. After a few days of exercise withdrawal, he began to become irritable and fidgety.

"So I figured, 'Since I can't run for a little while until this gets better, maybe I'll try swimming," he said. "Or maybe I'll get a bicycle and see what I can do with that.' At first, I had difficulty just swimming the length of the pool, but eventually that increased. Then I bought the bike and within a few weeks I fell off and broke my collarbone!

"That was late 1981. A few weeks later a friend said, 'Gee, now that you're into swimming, biking, and running, why don't you consider entering this thing called the 'Ironman Triathlon.' I said, 'What in the world is that?' We looked it up and found that it consisted of a 2.4-mile ocean swim, a 112-mile bike ride, and a 26-mile run. I figured since I could do all of those things, I'd give it a try."

Norton's first Ironman was February 6, 1982. It was a match made in heaven.

"I remember it well," he said. "It was just shortly after I had broken my collarbone, so I had to swim the entire 2.4 miles in a breast stroke because I couldn't get my left arm above my shoulder. Then I got on the bike. And, of course, I was a fairly good runner in those days, so I finished the first one in something under 17 hours. That was not only my first Ironman, that was the first of six times I was the oldest finisher. And that important bit of trivia and a dollar bill will get you a cup of coffee in some restaurants!"

Norton has continued to run the triathlons, but none attracted more attention than his second, in October 1983. ABC television discovered that he was the oldest competitor and their cameras followed him around the entire course.

"I didn't think much about it until ABC televised the race in February of the following year and gosh!—there were Norton and Betty on national TV!" he said. "That's when Betty became a national TV star overnight. That was a lot of fun—particularly the aftermath—because I got calls from all over the country."

Once the following year, Norton was in a store where the '83 Ironman was being rebroadcast on various television sets. He was watching the telecast when, suddenly, the announcers began to talk about him.

"They said, 'Here comes 65-year-old Norton Davey.' A couple of the shoppers kind of gasped and said, 'My gosh, that guy is 65!' And I couldn't resist saying, 'Yeah, he's crazy.'

"When they turned around to see who was speaking, they said, 'Hey, that's you!' That was fun—I'm a bit of a ham, I guess."

Like most addicts, Davey is at a loss to explain his affinity for the grueling—some would say nearly suicidal—Ironman Triathlons.

"Betty says it's because I like it," he said. "And I do! It's become something I look forward to every year, and I just hope they'll continue to let me enter each year and that each year I will be able to finish.

"Under the category of Very Important Trivia, I've started nine Ironman competitions, finished eight, and have been the oldest finisher six times. So in 1992 I'm going back for the 10th time. Jim Ward is about a year older, so when he finishes, he's the oldest finisher."

Fortunately for Norton, he has two very important "enablers" in his exercise-compulsive life: his wife, Betty, and his doctors.

"I was fortunate in picking the right gal 50 years ago," he said, "and I'm very fortunate in that Betty is supportive of what I do. She's my coach. I do work with another chap whom I consider my coach, but I consider Betty my coach at home. She's always been very supportive of this, I suppose, because she's noticed what it has done for me as far as my physical fitness is concerned. It has kept me in good health.

"She has been reluctant to travel to some of the local races any more simply because we've traveled so much in the past all over the world, and she has so many activities here in Leisure Village that she'd prefer to stay here. But I can count on her to go to Hawaii with me for a couple of weeks each year. And I'd be lost over there without her because she's not only mentally and morally supportive, she's just there all around the racecourse checking out other people, telling me where I stand. But the single greatest thing is that she looks after my diet. She feeds me well and we know what is good for us."

Betty, incidentally, is also in excellent physical condition, though she's never been tempted by the triathlons. She regularly participates in aerobics, and works out on the couple's stationary bike, rowing machine, and cross-country ski machine.

Additionally, both Norton's family doctor and his physicians through Continental have been supportive of his Ironman activities. They've also had a part in creating Norton's rigorous exercise routine and pre-Ironman Triathlon workout schedule.

"Training for the Ironman, I run four to six hours per day, six days a week, for three or four months," Norton said. "Then there is a tapering off after the Ironman.

"After that, I generally take it easy there for a few months, but I don't get out of shape—I just don't concentrate as much on the training regimen. Then I start again about June and work hard at that point."

In January, Norton begins running seriously once again, but cuts down on the hours spent on the bike or in the pool. This is in preparation for his *other* favorite event—the Catalina Marathon.

"We have a little island off the coast of California called Catalina that has no level part of it, except right at (the town of) Avalon," he said. "It's nothing but hills and mountains, not high mountains, but it's still pretty hilly. Each year since 1978 they have had the Catalina Marathon, which consists of running from one part of the island to finish in Avalon. It has become almost as attractive and as much fun for me as the Ironman simply because it is one heck of a challenge.

"Unfortunately, I've watched my times deteriorate over the years—that's one problem of getting old. I shouldn't say getting old: we're just not as young as we once were. I look forward to the Catalina and it comes in March each year. Those are usually the only two big events I'll do anymore, although occasionally, if there is a marathon in between somewhere, I'll enter. And I do enter a lot of smaller races."

Not that Norton's demanding schedule has been accomplished without cost. He admits that the sheer wear and tear of the Ironman and the marathons occasionally take their toll.

"Before I started running and doing triathlons, I didn't have nearly as many physical injuries as I have now," he said. "Any time I don't have an injury, I count my blessings. I know I'm in between injuries and I try to keep it that way. The injuries, particularly from running, are just legion—they're always there. I am, at this moment, slowly recovering from a stress fracture of about a month ago that I thought, initially, would knock me out of the 1992 Ironman. It'll slow down my running time, but it is coming back."

That physical pounding is partially compensated for by the fact that Norton has been uncommonly illness-free since he began running seriously.

"Since then, my health has been really good," he said. "My mother lived to be 91, so I guess I was blessed with good genes. But since I started running, I've had very few illnesses, save for the illnesses of old age—and they're no big deal.

"I do believe, in fact I'm firmly convinced, that this physical activity either slowed down the onset of middle age—or at least it has almost eliminated it. Without it, I would have, quite likely, probably had some other injuries."

Not that he could do it alone, either. Betty is in charge of the Davey diet, whether Norton is training for the Ironman or just lounging around the house, plotting future marathons and mountain climbs.

"We've always eaten moderately," he said. "Raising four kids, we would have meat just about every night because that was what we thought they needed back then to grow up. We always ate well, but they were balanced meals. As the kids slowly left home and there were just the two of us and I slowly got into this physical fitness thing, we found out that we not only didn't care for meat as much, but we just didn't eat it. Now we eat meat around two or three times per week and sometimes even less. And we'd prefer to go very heavy on vegetables, fruits, and pastas.

"More and more we're finding we're probably better off without meat. If we hadn't gotten in there and proven it, I don't think we would have believed that we could do this kind of training on a practically meatless diet."

This makes it sound like Norton is a single-minded obsessive-compulsive, that triathlons and marathons are the sole focus of his life. That's not true. He has other interests—like heavy-duty mountain-climbing.

"Prior to my climb of Kilimanjaro, I hiked up to the Mount Everest base camp in Nepal at about 18,300 feet," he said happily. "Several years ago I tried Mount Aconcagua in Argentina, the highest point in South America at 22,834 feet. I flunked that one and will not try it again. It was just too tough for me.

"There are two other things that I aspire to in this world that I am convinced I will not make: I won't make the summit of McKinley (Denali) in Alaska—simply because I don't like cold weather that well. The other thing is, as much as I will try, I don't think I will finish the Ironman in the daylight."

OK, so maybe Norton *is* a little single-minded. At least competing in the Ironman isn't some sort of religious experience.

Is it?

"I don't see any spiritual, religious drive to it," he said. "I suppose, deep down underneath, I count my blessings, if you will, that I am able to do this. And I recognize that somewhere there is a Supreme Being who is looking after me and taking care of me. But is He helping me to finish the Ironman Triathlon? I don't know. I think much more in down-to-earth ways.

"I do know that I find that training for the Ironman Triathlon is the greatest way I know to fight off the onset of middle age—or old age—depending how you look at it."

Norton said it is not uncommon for a young person to approach him at the Ironman Triathlons and ask him for his secret of longevity. He says it is no secret.

"I suggest to them that at *that* point he (or she) start exercising, if he is not already doing it," Norton said, "but do it slowly. If he intends to do it competitively, he should certainly get a complete physical examination because he might have some unknown underlying problems that would indicate he should *not* be doing this.

"If he has already hit the age of 30–40, I would caution him before he got too heavily hooked or committed to it that he balance things out. I have the greatest respect for triathletes that age, those that really know how to train."

But sometimes, serious training and having a life outside the triathlons are mutually exclusive. Norton says to excel in the Ironman Triathlon often means giving less attention to other parts of an athlete's life.

"First, you must train and train hard, which means many hours a day," he said. "Second, most athletes are working full-time, presumably, unless they're retired. You need to be gainfully employed to support an expensive habit like this one. And third, they're trying to keep a family together.

"If any one individual can combine those three things, I have the greatest admiration for him. I could not have done it back then. For one, I was so very devoted to my family while they were growing up that I wouldn't have wanted to take that much time away from them. And secondly, my occupation in helping run Continental Airlines often required anywhere from 60–80 hours a week. Therefore, that left no time for training.

"I could not have gotten into the triathlon business until after I had retired, although I did start running before then. But that kind of running didn't require nearly the dedication the triathlon requires."

If you're *still* interested in competing in the triathlon, Norton says you need to seriously consider your goals in life. *If* you can juggle training, work, and family, he says, by all means, go for it.

"Anybody who can do that, I admire," he said, "and we do have some great triathletes who can, men and women. But then there are many who cannot. Maybe they've lost a family along the way, or their work has suffered."

If someone is still willing to take the chance to become a world-class triathlete, Norton says there are a number of excellent books on training for the Ironman. But book-learning alone may not be enough.

"To become dedicated, that comes totally from within," he said. "How much *is* a man or woman dedicated to this matter of competition? I have run into many great triathletes who are splendid athletes, but who are not competitively motivated. They're not willing to go that additional mile running or swim those additional yards or bike those additional ten miles."

Davey said his goal now is not merely to register a respectable finish and win his age bracket, his sole purpose for entering either a marathon or an Ironman is to win.

"There are those who don't feel that way. There are many who philosophically feel (that) just to finish is enough," he said. "I guess I don't have the physical make-up to understand that."

Consequently, while Norton enjoys running/swimming/biking against younger athletes, he doesn't like *competing* against them.

"If I do do well in a triathlon, I like to have some recognition for it," he said. "I cannot compete against what I call 'the 60-year-old kids.' Years ago, I was one of them, but I'm not now. And when I have to enter a triathlon or a marathon that doesn't recognize there are 70-year-old and older athletes, that means I'm competing against these younger guys.

"Still, I enjoy it because I can beat some of them. It gets back to the thing (that) when I do something well, I like to have some personal recognition for it. That's part of the ham in me that likes the notoriety, the stroking at the end, to have a guy of the stature of Al Michaels say, 'And here comes 74-year-old Norton Davey... ' Now *that* sounds pretty good!"

What's ahead for Norton Davey? Frankly, he's not sure.

"I guess the future is uncertain at our age," he said. "We don't know whether we'll be around for one year or 20 years. Hopefully, Betty and I will live for many years. And, kind of selfishly, I hope she will outlive me. I'm not a particularly emotional guy I don't think, but on the other hand, it will be pretty tough to think about life without her. But she's in excellent health, so I think she will.

"On the other hand, can I continue to do it? Who knows? I guess we have to go back 20 years ago when who would have thought that a 74-year-old man could even enter, much less finish, an Ironman Triathlon? So who's to say we couldn't be doing it at age 85—in 10 years from now. I fully intend to enter every year, if I can.

"There are some definite drawbacks. The chances of injury are greater each year, either through trauma (a crash on a bike) or overuse. I remember I had a bad crash at a race in the Midwest two months before the Ironman, and as a result I was unable to finish it. It was too much to recover from a broken collarbone. It just took much longer."

It's also a matter of record that Norton takes much longer to complete the triathlon each year as well. Even a quick glance at his finishing times over the past 10 years reveals that he slows down about 20 seconds per mile per year.

"That's simply a matter of not being able to draw enough oxygen into the tissues to make them go like they used to," Norton said. "The muscles are saying, Hey, I need more oxygen—I'm not getting it. We try our darnedest to overcome that, but the body says no.

So, what's the bottom line, F. Norton Davey? How long will you continue to push your 74-year-old body to its outermost limits?

"Until I die," he said firmly. "Gee whiz—I'm going to be doing these things as long as I can qualify, as long as the Ironman will let me enter, as long as the marathons will let me.

"From my standpoint, I think the greatest way for me to go would be when I'm doing an Ironman Triathlon at age 88. 'He just collapsed on the highway,' they'll say. What a way to go!"

Chapter 8

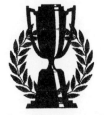

Bill Dunlap

MOUNT CALM, TEXAS—Folks say you have to put a rock in William "Bill" Dunlap's pocket to keep him from blowing away in a stiff, Texas wind. Bill looks like all the drug-store cowboys *wish* they could look. Lean and leathery, grizzled and gracious, with a pair of flinty eyes that look as if they could bore through steel.

At 78, Bill ropes calves on weekends for money. He ropes calves during the week for exercise. He ropes calves at night by lantern light for fun.

He's one of the top ropers in the National Old Timers Calf Roping Association, having won numerous individual ropings and, in 1985, the association's overall title.

To watch him and his horse burst out of the chute, arena dirt spraying like a wave behind them, rope whipping overhead, is to see a rare snippet of the Old West, an authentic fragment of a long-lost piece of Americana.

Bill hee-haws at the suggestion. It's just ropin', he patiently explains. Nothing romantic or artistic about it.

But to see Bill Dunlap and his horse work as a single unit is poetry in motion.

"I was raised near Hubbard, in Hill County, Texas," Bill drawled. "I was born August 25, 1914, on a farm. We had plow mules, 'walking busters.' We chopped and picked cotton.

"My daddy wouldn't even let me ride a horse. He didn't know I practiced roping on the mules—I'd rope our milk cow with a grass rope when I was 20 years old. I was born to rope.

"My daddy said, when I was a little kid, I'd go to the barn and take a rope rein and make a little loop in it—I was born to rope. Daddy took that and whupped me with it! He didn't want me to rope, he didn't want me to have a horse.

"From 1945 on, I farmed with mules on my farm south of Mount Calm. I had a plow mare I roped goats on when I was 28. I never had liked to rope goats. But I would do it anyway."

Along the way, he married Lillian (universally called Jimmie) and the couple had three children, two boys and a girl.

Bill was nearly 31 before he got his first horse.

During World War II, he helped organize the first rodeo club in Mount Calm.

"The first rodeo I was ever in I borrowed two horses and three-headed (roped and tied) three calves," he said. "I made the average time on three calves with twenty-something other ropers in the rodeo! There was a three-dollar entry fee for three.

"I've been roping ever since."

But most Central Texas farmer/ranchers barely eke out a hard-scrabble existence working dawn to dark, leaving little time for "foolishness" like calf roping. In time, Bill turned to horse-shoeing to augment his income.

"I farmed from 1945, but I've been shoeing horses for a living," he said. "Well, I take that back. In 1949, I got a job on a ranch for six years, but I still shoed horses. The man finally asked me to quit because I was shoeing horses at night, and on Saturday and Sunday on my days off.

"I'd shoe them at night with lights. I shoed a horse in Groesbeck one time by lantern light. I'd been shoeing horses and working in a blacksmith's shop, but it got to where you couldn't make a living doing it. When you're shoeing horses for three dollars, you ain't gonna make much."

Even after his so-called retirement—"I still do as much or more work than the average man"—a few years ago, Bill continues to shoe horses for friends and neighbors, mostly to pay the entrance fees to calf ropings.

"Sometimes I shoe three or four a week now," he said. "Not a whole lot. I don't look for them. A man called me yesterday and asked if I'd put two shoes on a mare. When I got down there, I said, 'You need all four on there.' So I went and shod her all around.

"I used to make them with the fire. We didn't have the ready-made shoes like you can buy now. It would take me nearly as long to build a fire and fit the shoes as it would to put them on."

In 1963, Bill built a pen on his small ranch with everything necessary to practice calf roping.

"I keep calves there year-round," he said. "I've roped twice this week. You can't rope enough. Calves have always been my favorite thing to rope. I used to team rope a little but I didn't really care for it. My boy likes team ropin'.

"I wasn't ever financially able to join the rodeo professionally. You've got to have money to do that."

Still, he displayed a natural gift for roping. When work on the farm would allow and he was between shoeing jobs, Bill would sometimes enter small Texas rodeos. And win.

"When I was 40, I won the Teague Rodeo with a low 10 seconds," he said. "But that was 38 years ago. I've won a few small jackpots by tying 'em down in nine seconds.

"I remember some boys in Waco that just about quit back when I was in my 40s. I'd spot 'em five seconds and beat 'em! They wouldn't let me in the pot unless I carried five with me! And I still beat 'em with a five-second handicap."

By the time Bill was financially able to rope regularly and had the time to do it, he was past the time he could have competed in professional rodeo.

But at 70 he discovered the National Old Timers Calf Ropers Association. He was on it like a duck on a June bug.

"I've been roping with them now for the past seven or eight years," Bill said. "When I started roping at 70, I was roping with the 65-year-olds. Now I'm roping with the 71-and-up age group. I just roped against a man who turned 71 last month, and I'm 78."

Bill has won three championship belt buckles for calf roping. His favorite memory is of the time he won the Old Timers Rodeo finals in Seguin, Texas, in 1985.

"I had a hip that had been tyin' up on me that year," Bill recalled. "I couldn't walk. I'd walk a couple hundred yards and I couldn't get back. So I went to a chiropractor because I was fixing to go to the Seguin finals.

"But that chiropractor said, 'Aw, Bill, you need to quit ridin' them horses.' I told him, 'When I quit ridin' them horses is when I can't get on them. I've got the Seguin finals coming up in a couple weeks.' And I went. I went and won that one for ropin' six calves."

In 1991, Bill was again in the finals, even though the category was 65-and-up. The eventual winner was a cowboy who had just turned 65.

"I don't have a chance against a man roping at age 65," he snorted. "Still, I messed around and missed my first one—you gonna miss one now and then, everybody's gonna miss one. It cost me a buckle and I was entered in the 65-and-up category!

"Come up the last calf and I had 23 seconds to win that buckle, but the calf got to kickin' on me and I went to 24 seconds.

"Last week I fumbled one up while I was tyin' him down and got a 15—should have had a 13. 'Nother man won it with a 13. I was second. That's the way it goes."

Calf roping is not a sport for the faint of heart or the weak of knee. Bill's willowy frame is deceptively strong. When Bill ropes a calf, it *knows* it's been roped!

"They tell me that's what keeps me going—my ropin'," he said, "but roping ain't all I do. I exercise five and six days a week on a concrete floor in the den. I've got a thing called a 'gut-buster' (a spring-resistance exerciser). I lay flat on my back and pull it 50–60 times to my stomach. You don't see many 78-year-olds who can do that, do you?

"I've got a pole in this den and I grab it and I squat down. Ten years ago, I couldn't squat down like that and get up. Now I do squats and keep my knees limber. I started about six years ago. My knees got so bad, I had to. A horse pulled me down 20 years ago and hurt my knee on the pavement. I had to quit roping for a while, it hurt me so bad. I couldn't sit; I couldn't even drive with it. I'd move it to the left and it would jump out of place! Now it doesn't get out of place.

"And I've got a stationary bicycle I ride at least one-to-three miles, three or four times a week. And I've got a regular bike I ride down the road."

The rest of the time you can find Bill out in his pen on horseback, practicing his roping on a dummy. And usually at full speed.

As a result, Bill says that he's in better shape now than he's been in five years—or more.

"See, I'm more limber now than before," he said. "I get flat on my back and do sit-ups. I do 30 sit-ups now. When I first started, I couldn't do five. You know those back problems I had back in '85? Once I started doing my exercise, it didn't bother me no more. Sit-ups took care of all my back problems.

"When I first started with that gut-buster, this knee would go on me after 10. Now I can go at least 30 times."

If his exercise routine sounds exceptional, his diet is even more so. Bill says he simply doesn't eat.

"I *don't* eat," he said flatly. "I got no appetite. You know, a lot of people eat all the time. I eat a bowl of Wheaties for breakfast and I won't want nothing until three o'clock—and even then I'm not hungry.

"My wife says, 'You don't eat enough.' I say, 'Well, if you're not hungry, why should you eat?'

"My little grandson laughs at me because I like fried eggs and sausage for supper. Now *that* tastes good. He says, 'Aw, Grandpa, that's breakfast.' I can eat anything when I want to, though."

Strange as it sounds, it's hard to argue with facts. There just isn't a whole lot of Bill Dunlap there, even though he stands nearly six feet tall. Even in the late afternoon, he doesn't cast much shadow.

About every five years, Bill will see a doctor. Once it was for strep throat. Another time it was a kidney stone. Then about 10 years ago, Bill had "sort of a heart attack." Or something.

"I got too hot running some calves afoot—trying to pen them. I got to sweatin'," he said. "My eyes began to blur. They brought me to Waco to the doctor. I hadn't been to him much. I told him: 'When you feel like I do, why do you want a checkup? I feel like a million dollars. Just let me get on my horse, get out in my pen, and run me four, five calves. I'll feel great.'

"Worst thing was when I went to the emergency room and the nurse took my blood pressure—she never did tell me how low it was. She said, 'It's too low to check.'

"They wanted me to stay in the hospital, but by then I felt like I do now: good. So I said, 'I'm going to see my granddaughters play softball. Sorry.' The doctor said what I had was a flutter."

Bill had to admit that he'd never asked the few doctors he *has* seen if they think calf roping is such a good idea for a 78-year-old.

On the other hand, his wife Jimmie has made no bones about her opposition to the sport—and Bill's participation in it.

"She's just never liked my calf roping," he said. "She never has. I've never heard her say, 'I hope you win' or 'I'm glad you won' as long as I've been going. I won the Seguin buckle and all she said was, 'You can buy one just like that for $75 to $100!'"

It's pretty obvious that Jimmie's icy glare isn't going to get Bill out of calf roping. It's as much a part of him as his horses. And, like most true cowboys, Bill can wax eloquent on his horses. But no horse has ever matched up to Frank. In Bill's unbiased estimation, Frank was the greatest horse that ever lived. Bill rode Frank for more than 20 years.

"Heck, I roped some calves on him when he was 28," he said. "He hadn't had a saddle on him in a year. He never liked to run no long ways in the arena; he knew there wasn't no money at the other end of the arena. But he'd go in that chute every time I asked him—half a dozen times if I asked him.

"A TV cameraman once filmed me ropin' calves on Frank three months before he died, when he was 31. And he did it! I got two of the slowest calves I had—and they wasn't slow. I rode him with just a halter—I couldn't find his bridle. I roped 'em both down. He wanted to run some more! That was the last time I had a saddle on him.

"Three months later he lay down and died. I told that cameraman, 'I'm glad we run them calves on him that day.'

"I put a marker where I buried Frank."

If this sounds like a man at peace with the world, you're right. Give Bill a bowl of Wheaties, a roping pen, a couple of feisty calves, a good horse, and all's right with the world.

"I wake up lookin' for tomorrow," he said. "You don't know if you're even going to be here today. One man I knowed since I was in high school. He'd had heart problems. They found him dead one day this week pinned under his tractor. They figure he had the heart attack and got off. The man was a farmer for 60 years.

"Another man, a friend of mine up in Hubbard, had a heart attack under a shredder. If I have heart problems, I reckon I'll quit."

A newspaper reporter once asked the president of Bill's calf roping association about Bill. He said, "The bond among horse and man and calf is a strong one. If Bill couldn't rope, he'd be dead. It's the horse out there in the pen that pulls the man out of bed. It may sound crazy, but it's the truth."

Bill replies, "Like the man said, when I quit ropin', I'll be dead. Now my wife said I better quit sayin' that. So I told her, 'OK, I'll quit when I can't get on my horse.'"

Don't expect *that* to happen any time soon. He's up at daybreak, nearly every day, practicing his roping alone.

Incidentally, one of Bill's sons has turned into a pretty fair roper, too. "He just don't like to get up early and rope with me," Bill said solemnly. "I don't like to lay in bed; I *can't* lay in bed.

"Let's see: I got no appetite and I don't sleep none. They say an old man sleeps like a baby. That's right, too: I sleep two hours and wake up and cry! I feel good, so I guess I get enough sleep.

"And, you know, I *still* never get hungry."

Chapter 9

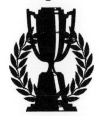

Phil Guarnaccia

BREA, CALIFORNIA—*50 Plus* magazine once had this to say about Phil Guarnaccia: "Guarnaccia is a pussycat in a lion's body. Soft-spoken but iron-willed, he is probably the most physically fit man over 50 in America."

But here's an even better picture of Phil. For the past 20 years, he's had a standing offer: match my five-and-a-half-hour daily workout and I'll pay you $10,000 cash. Two hundred competitors tried and failed. In 1984, a crew from the television show *That's Incredible!* took a then-60 Phil up on his offer. But when they arrived, they brought three bodybuilders whose *combined* ages weren't much more than 60.

For the next 11 grueling hours, under the arid white heat of the television cameras, Phil defeated them one after the other. Finally, late in the evening, he took his turn on the 120-pound barbell for the Roman Curls, placed it behind his head, and began to do sit-ups off the end of a bench.

"Guarnaccia's stomach rippled and twitched and then burned like never before," reported *Cyclist* magazine. "Late in the night, he finished off the last challenger. A month later he reluctantly checked into a hospital with a torn abdominal wall."

Shortly after that—convalescence be damned—Phil entered yet another bicycle race. This time he shredded his stomach muscles so finely that surgeons were forced to weave a Dacron mesh to knit the tattered filaments. Three months later he was racing again.

Now *that's* a good Phil Guarnaccia story!

But this man who holds a host of cycling championship records, not just in his masters' age groups, but in the tough 40-Plus age bracket, is just *full* of stories like that.

Even his early days read like a latter-day Horatio Alger tale.

His parents were immigrants from Sicily, who arrived in East Boston during the Depression with $25 and not a word of English between them. They worked hard in the factories so that young Phil could go to school, which he did—usually taking different routes up dark back alleys each day to avoid getting beaten up by the neighborhood bullies.

In time, Phil had had enough. He built a home gym on the tiny patio and created barbells out of cement blocks. According to *Cyclist* magazine, his father didn't approve:

"He said, 'Education is power.' 'Might be so,' I said, 'but I'm getting tired of getting beaten up.' For me, it was a question of survival."

Phil also survived four years in the Navy during World War II. He trained as an electrician, but spent many of his off-duty hours studying bodybuilding and reading about weight-lifting competitions. After the war, he threw himself into both.

"Following my discharge from the Navy, I got into bodybuilding and a weight-lifting routine," he said. "I followed that for some nine years and won the Mr. California competition."

Phil was a featured cover boy in a dozen bodybuilding magazines. At 5'8", and 205 pounds, he had an incredible chest and arms, equal to any steroid-enhanced competitor of today.

"Then one day in 1953, I was invited to go out for a bicycle ride with the San Francisco Wheelmen, a bicycle club," he said. "At that time, I weighed around 205 pounds of fairly solid muscle. I agreed."

The trip was a day's outing: a quick 26-mile jaunt to build up an appetite for lunch.

"We were on a ride of 13 miles up some sort of grade, and within one mile I had two cyclists pushing me up the hill!" he said. "And I had just won a title called 'Mr. Physical Fitness!' I honestly felt I was in top, physically fit, shape.

"But to my disappointment, I was forced to go back to the drawing board to find out what I had been doing for nine years that made me so physically unfit when I'd won these various titles!"

The experience changed his life. With the same single-minded obsession with which he had studied bodybuilding, Phil now studied physical fitness and health.

"After a lot of studying, I finally made a change in my training routine, which involved aerobic and anaerobic training and getting rid of 40-odd pounds of weight," he said.

"Bodybuilding is very incomplete," he told *Cycling*, "it's the muscles that you can't see that are important."

And the beautiful, massive physique he'd spent thousands of hours sculpting in the gym? He discovered that it was nothing more than a superficial "aesthetic"—what he called a "suit of armor encasing a neglected heart."

The new books on physiology gave him a new routine, but Phil wanted something more. He tried various competitive, athletically oriented-sports before returning to the one that had started it all: cycling.

"I've been cycling for 35–36 years," he said. "I feel today that I have the combination of bulk, which is extremely essential—I still subscribe to bodybuilding and weight-lifting magazines—and fitness I want.

"You know, it is amazing to see these bodies which are now steroid-formed and assisted and I just think it is hurting the general public more than anything else. It is such a simple message: get in good shape on your own and maintain yourself and you can achieve a quality of life that's unbelievable."

Thirty-five years of daily five-and-a-half-hour workouts—including a daily 50-mile bicycle ride—have not diminished Phil's initial enthusiasm.

"It is rather amazing that the further I got into this physical thing, the more interesting it became," he said. "I'm still training today for several reasons: I honestly feel I haven't even approached my potential. It is amazing because most people feel that, as they enter into their older years, they should slack off. But it is just the opposite! You should increase your training.

"It's just like a brand new automobile. You can take that brand new automobile and abuse the hell out of it and it will run until one day, it will stop. For no reason. You say, 'I just can't understand this car. It has been running for so many years and now it is all gone.' The body is pretty much the same way. You can abuse your young body and it will survive the younger years. But as you approach the older years, you've got to take care of it. The place to take care is during your younger years. You've got to build that foundation and, if you do that, there should be no reason why you can't get into a quality life."

Within months, Phil's regimen began to pay dividends, both in his personal fitness and on the cyclists' circuit.

"At the time I started out, there was no masters' division," he recalled, "so I was forced into racing with the Class A, B, and C riders—'A' being at the top of the list. Actually, that was a blessing because it really forced you into a line of training so that if you just finished in the first 10, *that* was an achievement!

"While there's nothing like first place, nevertheless it brought me to a level of fitness so high that, eventually, when they started a masters' class for ages 40 and over, after years of cycling with the Class A riders—and even winning a few races there—stepping into the masters' class was relatively easy at the time!"

Fortunately, Phil said that as the years rolled by and as awareness of fitness and health rose, so the quality of riders in the older categories rose with it.

"The 1992 masters' class today is a very viable class," he said. "But if you looked at it 10 years ago, it wasn't. So victories came relatively easy because of the level of training prior to that. Today, if you're going to win a masters' class, you've got to do your homework! So the last five years, it has been progressively tougher, regardless of the age rating they have set.

"So I've been racing in the 40 and 45-plus category for many, many years. And today they have classes all of the way up to 80 years old and some of these 80-year-old guys are coming out of the woodwork!"

Today there have been so many races and so many victories that Phil says they tend to blur together in his mind. He has a room full of trophies and awards.

"Still, certain races stand out over the years," he said. "Most of them you promptly forget because they are routine races. I honestly feel that the first state title I won was quite rewarding back in the mid-'70s. I remember thinking, 'Gee, that was such a great race, I don't think I could ever do that again.' But it is amazing that, once you hit that level, you start looking at other levels.

"Next, I think about my first national title in Florida in the early 1980s. And I thought, 'I don't believe I could ever exceed this!' The level seemed to increase and here it is, nine national titles later, and I'm still going after them. It is amazing because each one is a new adventure!

"Of course, now comes the world title. I haven't had the time to venture over to Europe, but that's on the books as well."

The training routine required to maintain that level of cycling success is more than a little intimidating. Phil's daily workout has an epic quality about it.

He rises early, has breakfast, reads the newspaper, then goes into his gym. Phil has his own studio in his home. It was once located at his office (PG Electrical Contracting) in a separate warehouse with 4,000 square feet of gym space—with gym equipment, showers, and lockers for employees and clients. But he was forced to move it home because only one employee ever used the gym.

"First, I'll go to a full-body routine of all major muscle groups," he said. "I'll finish it off on a stationary bike for one hour. That takes me to the first part of the morning. After lunch, I'll check on my office and see what's happening there. And then I go for an afternoon ride of approximately 50 miles. I average about 300 miles a week on the bicycle, usually two and a half hours a day. I do six days on the workout, seven days on the bike.

"I have what I refer to as a summer routine and a winter routine. Of course, the intensity of the winter routine reduces time on my bicycle. As the racing season approaches, the intensity increases. The only difference is the intensity of the workout. As I get to the competitive season, my intensity increases. As the season ends, the intensity decreases. The workouts remain the same. I don't miss many meals and I don't miss many workouts. I eat year round and I train year round. It is part of my life and it is part of maintenance—and it should be."

Phil believes that diet is as important to his health and fitness regimen as the physical workout. New studies are being released almost daily that appear to back him up.

"My diet has changed over the years as I'm learning more about my body and more about what it needs," he said. "The sad thing about this is that it takes pretty much a lifetime to acquire that. My eating habits today are entirely different than they were 30–35 years ago. It is surprising how little food I need to survive. Just a handful of food will do after all of those years of stuffing all of those foods down. It takes a lot of energy to process that much food through your body—energy that you could be using for something else. So, my eating habits over the years have changed considerably.

"Today, I just eat basic foods that comprise approximately: 70 percent carbohydrates, possibly 10–12 percent protein at the most, and I try to keep it under 10 percent fat."

In recent years, Phil has become more and more convinced that the true culprit in American diets is fat. His ultimate goal is to eliminate *all* fat from his diet.

"I want zero fat," he said. "I find that by trying to eliminate fat completely, I still get too much. There's so much fat in the food to begin with. So, if I go for the 0 percent fat, *no* fat at all—and that includes the entire family of dairy products—I find that I'm getting more than enough fat. So I'll increase my carbos up to maybe 80 percent and my protein a few more, and that's it. And I'm *still* getting too much fat. Just because the foods are processed that way, you cannot avoid it and what is there is more than ample.

"As you become older, it is more important to cut down on fat because the metabolic functions in your body slow down and if you increase your fat intake, you're just going to get fat! You're going to add more fat to fat!"

Additionally, Phil says he only gets a small amount of his protein from meats.

"I'm not a vegetarian 100 percent, although I do limit my meat intake to chicken and fish," he said. "Red meat I have just pretty much eliminated. I've experimented with myself over the years, and the meat really slows me down. It slows me down in the processing and digesting of the food, as well as my performance on the bicycle. In the course of the year, I just might have a steak now and then, but only because that's the only thing on the menu. As a rule, I eat either chicken or fish.

"I honestly feel in the nutritional end of it, which is so important, I would say basically this is where you start. And then you can add the exercise to it to complete the package. But you better eat right as well as train right."

Today, at age 68, Phil has become something of a fitness guru, an indefatigable crusader on positive lifestyle choices.

"It's rather amazing—and while I can only refer to the country I've been born and raised in—but it is absolutely amazing that there are some people here who feel that to get up and go to the bathroom they've accomplished something at that age," he said. "And yet, most of the people I know in their 80s are running marathons and riding their bicycles 25 miles per day. And this is such a natural thing for them.

"I was asked this question years ago: 'Will this extend my life?' I would say, 'No, the quality will rise, but the extension of life will not.' Ask me the same question today, and I can guarantee you that it will add 10 years of good living—or more!—to your life if you will follow some basic routine. It's very simple. Most people hardly miss any meals each day, but they sure miss their workout."

Strangely enough, Phil says that despite the current research, he has found entrenched resistance to his message of wellness and fitness.

"Years ago, my doctors were not supportive," he said. "I train with doctors a lot and I have several relations (who) are doctors and I'm trying to keep them alive! The last person you want to listen to if you want to live longer is a doctor! They know nothing about nutrition or wellness! There are a few exceptions, but not many.

"Anyway, the doctors were not supportive of any kind of physical exercise back in the 1940s. When the war ended in 1945 and I got into serious training, the biggest objection I heard from doctors all of the time was, 'Phil, you don't want to train this hard because your heart is like a beach balloon and you'll have—what they referred to at that time—an athletic heart.' They said, 'You're just destroying yourself.'"

Today, of course, a heart enlarged—strengthened, actually—through exercise is an asset. A stronger heart pumps more blood per beat and works less at rest than the unconditioned heart.

"I've buried every one of the doctors that criticized my training in those early years," Phil said, "I'm still going, but they're not.

"The opinions today from the new doctors are very supportive of this type of training. There is an area of overtraining, but the mental aspects of that probably hurt more than the physical aspects of it. You just get stale and tired. That's curable by decreasing the workout somewhat—not stopping it!"

While most doctors have come around, Phil says that this level of fitness and health are harder still for many families to accept, much less embrace.

It's a subject Phil is intimately acquainted with. His wife Laura, a heavy smoker, died at age 45 of a brain hemorrhage brought on by chronic high blood pressure.

"I think that you're going to find a lot of trouble in that area," he said softly. "If you are a devoted trainer and a true, full-time champion, there's very little time left for family affairs. You will see a terrible negative effect on family life. I don't recommend this type of training I'm following to anyone.

"I certainly don't believe that a family man should go through this type of routine that I'm following. Certainly, most people have an hour a day. Or, you can close it down to 22 minutes a day, seven days a week, and still leave ample time for family life and all of the other social events you might want to go to and still maintain a pretty fair level of health. I think the average family man certainly can devote that type of time to it and still have time for his family.

"The big difference between competitive fitness and just plain health and fitness is that the former will take so much more time. The type of training I do will just almost cut your family out of it. I think you will find this true in any sport. If the level of training is top-notch, something else has to be sacrificed."

But there are other, less visible, health benefits to be gained. Phil says, for instance, that most of the common ailments that dog twentieth-century man have rarely plagued him.

"As far as general health is concerned, I don't think I've had three headaches in my life," he said. "And I feel cheated because I see everybody else having headaches, complaining about indigestion. I honestly feel I can eat cast-iron nuts and bolts. I digest food very well and very rapidly.

"I just feel good every morning and sometimes I wonder, 'How long can this go on?' I'm a little concerned about it—I'm concerned that I might wake up one morning and not feel right.

"I understand that, genetically, I'm gifted in that area: my father is still alive at 96 years old and he's still working out, and still driving a car. So, the genetics are fine and that's a major step in the right direction.

"But more importantly than that, I do follow a system of body maintenance on a day-to-day basis. I enjoy a level of health today that's not paralleled anywhere else, really."

People tend to notice things like that. Particularly after magazine or newspaper articles, middle-aged people shyly approach Phil and ask about *their* chances of achieving something even approximating his level of health and fitness.

"I've been approached this way a lot," Phil confirmed. "My approach to people who come into my home or come into my office in their 50s, people who never did anything up to that point, and now, suddenly, realize, 'Hey, I would like to get into some kind of exercise routine to improve my health,' is this: 'Fine. Let's find out basically what your foundation is at this point, and then go from there as far as what you are trying to achieve—and can achieve—starting late.'"

But what about those people who come up to you and say, "Phil, I want to get up to your level?"

"I'll say, 'I don't know if that's possible, because I started at 13 and I have that foundation—and you build on it just like a pyramid—and you've lost a lot of that," Phil said.

"You stand an excellent chance of getting to the level you have chosen. But you may have to settle for a lower level. But in any event, in any case, you *will* improve. Depend on it. It is well worth it. You will improve, there's no question about it. You're not going to hurt yourself, so the time spent on health is well spent."

Notice how Phil says "health" so much. It's a key word in his vocabulary, even more than "fitness" or "training."

"I say health because that's the number one issue here," he said. "The competitiveness and the champion this and the champion that is fine. But I'm training now to maintain or even improve my health."

One of the best ways to achieve that level of health, at any age, Phil believes, is to set goals.

"But they shouldn't be so high that you can't remotely achieve them, nor so low that they're too easy," he said. "They should be beyond fingertip reach. So when you reach that level, you push up even higher because continual failures are discouraging as well. You build health as you build anything: with progressive steps. You continue to build for that level.

"I've had doctors come back and tell me that when I approach 85, my strength level will be down to a 10-year-old's. This is so ridiculous. It *will* go down to a 10-year-old's if I do nothing up to age 85. I guarantee you that. Today I enjoy no more than a 15 percent loss in strength from the time I was the strongest. It's rewarding to be able to say that. I can do exactly what I did when I was 25 years old. That's 15 percent less—not 70 percent less."

There is still one more side to Phil Guarnaccia, one that is making waves in business magazines rather than health and fitness magazines.

Drawing on his expertise as an electrician, Phil founded PG Electrical Contracting in 1965, with himself as the sole employee. Today PG Electrical has 22 employees housed in 8,000 square feet of office and warehouse space in Brea.

Although PG Electrical has a fine reputation for contracting in the Los Angeles area, it's Phil's innovative health plan and incentive program that have caught the attention of businessmen everywhere.

"If you hire in, the first thing I do is take your pulse rate for about four or five days so I can come up with an average number," Phil said. "Now, reduce that average number by 10 percent. Assume you come in at 100 beats per minute and you reduce it to 90—I'll give you $1,000. The best part of all is this: if you keep it at 90 or lower, I'll continue to give you $1,000 annually, as long as you continue to do it. And there's only one way you're going to do that: progressively exercise to keep it down. Anybody, *anybody* can bring it down 10 percent just by walking a little, just by doing very simple things. And there's $1,000.

"Or if you have a weight problem, I will pay you for every pound you shed, the price of filet pound per pound. It might be five to six dollars per pound, or I'll it give it to you in meat. If you're a meat eater, I'll buy you a pound of filet mignon for every pound you lose. I will pay you for that."

That's not all. Phil pays all smokers at PG Electrical $500 to quit smoking.

"It's easy to fire people for smoking," he said. "You'll lose some good employees that way. Of course, you're going to lose them if they continue to smoke anyway! But $500—and this is a small company—for you to drop that cigarette. Some companies may give you $50 or $125 or something of that order—but this is $500 cash.

"I only add a couple of small stipulations. First of all, if you resume smoking, I want my $500 back. Secondly, I want the accrued interest that money would have brought in, had it been in my possession. I think that's a hell of a bargain."

Alas, it is the more general areas of physical fitness and health that seem to have stymied even the ever-resourceful Phil. When he had the fully equipped gym at PG Electrical, he offered every employee that worked out there four times a week his or her full hourly wage for that time—just for working out!

"A Class A electrician today demands $20–25 per hour," he said. "I would have paid them that for working out for a full hour every day on my time. But very few take me up on it.

"If they tell me they don't like the gym equipment, I say, 'Fine: park yourself a mile down the road and I'll pay you to walk to work!'

"It is very possible for each employee to pick up somewhere between $2,500 and $3,000 dollars per year. Just don't come into my office and ask for a percentage raise—unless you take advantage of that physical program first. That can pay you in two ways: you can earn real cash, and you're going to improve your level of health, which you couldn't buy anywhere."

It is an exciting, genuinely innovative program, one that has been examined by businessmen across the country. But

Phil grudgingly admits that, for the most part, it has been a failure. "The sad part of it is that I must be the poorest salesman in town," he said, "because I have less than two percent working out! I got to the point where I had to move all of the equipment out of there because I couldn't justify the expense of keeping it in the workplace." Phil even opened his facilities free of charge to Brea's police and fire departments—but the offer didn't generate a single regular user.

"Still, as far as I know, this is the only company of any size that does the things I do—and that includes the giants like General Motors, Westinghouse, and the oil companies."

There are other incentives, other similar programs at PG Electrical, but you get the picture.

In the end, Phil claims to be involved in PG Electrical Contracting only to the point of checking the bottom line each day.

"The numbers I'm interested in only answer the question, 'Are we in the red or in the black?'" he said. "If they're in the black, I'm not too interested. If they're in the red, I am. That's my involvement in the business.

"My interest now is focused on helping senior adults stay fit."

It's not an idle boast, either. In recent years, Phil has channeled his not-inconsiderable energy and resources into the looming health-care problem. He believes that health care will one day emerge as America's greatest individual crisis.

"My focus now in this country is that your health is your situation," he said. "I no longer can afford to try to improve your health, the system being what it is. So the responsibility for your health is yours.

"Forty percent of the people in hospitals today put themselves in there. It all goes back to day one. Our education system has to change. Learning how to take care of yourself is so important. A larger percentage of the population cannot afford medical care any longer. We've got to learn how to take care of ourselves so we don't need medical care. And we've got to educate people when they first get into kindergarten about the importance of health and fitness.

"I can design a program that's for very busy people. The first thing they say is, 'I don't have time.' That's a lot of baloney. When you're sick, you make the time to go to the doctor's office and then sit in that waiting room an hour and a half. You make that kind of time. But if people say they don't have 22 minutes a day, there's something wrong with them.

"The body is an extremely forgiving piece of machinery. If you treated your automobile like most people treat their bodies, it'd be a piece of junk in two and a half years. Just the amount of salt people consume would eat out the radiator!"

What's ahead for Phil Guarnaccia? He doesn't know. He won't even begin to guess. He can't see that far in the future.

"Because I've enjoyed a level of health that very few people even come close to, my plans are based on long-term achievements," he said. "I'm looking forward to the next 10–15 years.

"Now if my health were bad or failing, I would be a day-to-day man. But I'm not a day-to-day man, I'm a long-term, long-goal type of individual because I believe I'll be around at that time. And, more importantly, with a quality of health that I can enjoy."

Chapter 10

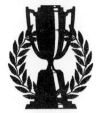

Joseph Hauser, Jr.

ODENTON, MARYLAND—Joseph Hauser, Jr., is pushing his souped-up Datsun 1600 roadster hard around the black-scarred track in Gainesville, Georgia. It's the 1992 Sports Car Club of America championship and Joe, who qualified with the fourth-fastest speed in his class, is looking good.

At 73, Joe's not only the oldest competitor, he's one of the most respected. After all, he's got 120 victories under his belt since 1969.

Joe sees an opening and shoots his Datsun through the gap. The leader is in sight. Suddenly, the car just ahead of him spins out, knocking both of them out of the race for good.

Rattled but unhurt, Joe storms from the car.

"Oh well," sighs Lois, his wife of 50 years. "There's always next year."

What's another year when you're 73 years young?

Or, as fellow competitor Randy Canfield once told *USA Today:* "He looks in his 70s and walks like his 70s, but he sure doesn't *drive* like his 70s."

But then, driving *something* has been Joe's life for nearly all of those 73 years.

As a farm boy growing up near Nashville, Kansas, Joe began driving the family tractors and trucks at age nine.

"Even on the farm I had my first car," he said. "And back then we didn't need driver's licenses—I got a Model T when I was about 14. I remember that it was even in my name! In Kansas you didn't need a driver's license. So I actually started driving cars and tractors at age nine to and from the fields. I've always been interested in driving.

"I was born and raised in the Depression, so I started late to high school and made it through high school in three years. I attended college for only six months before I went into the Army Air Corps in 1942, which is where I got into flying.

"I flew two missions during the war in Europe, came back on the Berlin Airlift, then did another tour of Europe. In the 24 years I was in the Air Force, we were in probably 12–15 different locations. We got shuffled around pretty much from 1945 until 1955, when we kind of settled down."

While stationed in Germany, Joe became familiar with what was called auto-cross.

"I did do a little hill-climbing and auto-cross in various parking lots and arena parking lots," he said. "That's where I got the real bug to race because the hill climbs in Germany were very interesting. They had speed events where you close off a hill and race up it. This was back in the late '50s and early '60s.

"As far as racing goes, I would have liked to have started before I did, but in the Air Force, that's really difficult when you move every two or three years. I really never got a chance until I was assigned to the Washington, D.C., area and we had a local chapter of an organization called the Sports Car Club of America."

In the years before Joe retired in 1965, he cross-trained into electronics—a skill that would serve him in good stead in the years ahead. He then worked for the government for another 16 years, before he retired for good in 1982 with 40 years of government service. ("That was enough.")

"It wasn't until 1964 that I got started in close-course racing," Joe said. "I've always been interested in mechanical things and, of course, especially in flying. Fortunately, I got a shot at both of them."

After his retirement, Joe threw himself into SCCA racing. The SCCA was begun right after World War II by a number of American car enthusiasts who returned home with English sports cars. Initially, the emphasis in sports car racing was on air fields and runways. Today it is a national organization that promotes what was once called "amateur racing," but is now generally called club racing.

"We race strictly for trophies, although some manufacturers give some sponsorship money," Joe said. "It's mostly gentleman-type racing and you support your own car. I build my own engine—that's part of my hobby. It's really a very time-consuming hobby! I figure I spend 100 hours working on the car for every one hour I spend on the track.

"The rules allow you to modify the car substantially and you're always trying to figure some way to make it go faster. There have to be rules that are laid down by the club. Otherwise people would spend fortunes to win a trophy."

The SCCA has two levels, regional and national. From 1964–69, Joe raced almost exclusively on the regional level. In 1969, he switched over to the national competition. Since that time he's won a whopping 120 races. But how many did he win on the regional level?

"I don't know," he admitted, "I never kept track of what I won there! I didn't start keeping records until I started racing on the national level."

National champions are settled in a seven-division shoot-out held each November in Gainesville, Georgia.

"It's an invitational thing," Joe said. "We race within our division and there are seven divisions. The top people at each race get points for first, second, third, and fourth. At the end of the season, the last qualifying races for the run-offs are the first weekend of September. The run-offs are around October 14–15. So we get four cars in each class, from seven divisions, and we have a real shoot-out!

"I've won four times in Gainesville. Unfortunately, I haven't won since 1982. I qualified on the pole position in 1992 and had a good shot at it. I just had a real good qualifying time, but I didn't really have the best car there. I should have finished second or third, but I spun out and finished fourth."

One of the things Joe likes about the SCCA is that there is no discrimination of any kind, neither of age, race, or sex.

"There is everybody from 18 to however old you can get—which is usually me!" he said with a laugh. "Sure, I have a ball racing against 18-year-olds. You get a lot of satisfaction out of competing with people that other people say have better reaction times.

"It's only by car class and the cars are classed by a competition board. They sit down every year and look at how the cars have run within their classes. If one kind of car is dominating, they do something to slow it down or move it up to the next higher class. The cars are kind of varied within classes, so they're classified by car potential."

Joe's Datsun 1600 is in the "G Production" class. He says that some of the various classes are not as well-populated now as they were 20 years ago, because some of the cars are getting older.

"The board hasn't moved any new cars in 'G,' so it is getting a little easier to win," Joe said. "But not at the run-off—those are the best cars in the division nationwide."

Interestingly enough, it was a classification dispute that led to the most memorable—and satisfying—race in Joe's long and storied career.

"Most race car drivers have pretty big egos—they have to spend all this money and time," Joe said. "And the one thing we like to do is win. Not long ago I had a different kind of car, an Austin-Healy, that the competition board saw fit to move from one classification to another, which I fought verbally and by letters. But I lost.

"So I went to one of the guys, wrote him a nasty note in a business letter, and told him I was going out and buying me a Datsun and I was going to win that class! I wasn't sure I could do it—but that's what I did! And *that* was the most satisfying race I ever won.

"Of course, you can guess what they did. They handicapped me the next time—they added 100 pounds to my car!"

Despite his spin-out in the most recent nationals, and despite more than two decades of racing in less-than-optimum conditions, Joe has never suffered a significant injury while racing.

"I have had a couple cars that I wrecked and didn't rebuild," he said, "but other than the time during one of my accidents where I saw a couple of stars, I haven't had any injuries."

That kind of track record is due to more than luck. Joe chalks it up to both experience and conditioning.

"Basically, I don't really give much emphasis to age," he said. "I think I'm as good a driver now as when I started in 1964 when I was 45 or 46. I find that my timing and my driving skills, which are part of what I judge myself by—since I run the same tracks, basically, every year—have gotten better and better over the years.

"Of course, the tires and cars have gotten a little better. I've got to admit your reactions do slow up a little, but I think because you keep practicing, it doesn't matter much. That's the thing: if I ever dropped out of racing, I don't think I could really come back for a while. It would take a while to get back to speed.

"I think flying helped—it teaches you to look ahead and think ahead. That's the big problem for a lot of people in race car driving. They don't see a problem coming up because they're looking only at a point just in front of their car. You've got to look ahead and plan what you're going to do."

As for the conditioning, Joe says every other year, each driver over the age of 40 is required to take a thorough, comprehensive physical that includes an EKG, because racing *is* both stressful and physically demanding.

"Steering a car isn't really hard or heavy, although my Datsun takes more effort than any of the older cars I had," he said. "Still, you have to be in pretty good physical shape because you have to run in any kind of weather, whether it is 95 or 100 degrees. And you have to wear double- or triple-layer no-burn suits, and you perspire a lot. So you have to be in fairly decent physical condition. Otherwise, you find towards the end—even though our races are only 30–40 minutes long—you find yourself getting pretty darn tired. I've tried to keep myself in good physical condition."

Joe's workout routine includes some walking and gardening, along with regular swimming sessions with his wife Lois.

"Mostly, I work on my own cars," he said, "but I've kept in pretty good shape. I've always been about 6 foot, 185 pounds. I try to eat moderately. When I was a kid, my parents were great ones for balanced meals. My dad saw that we had a couple vegetables, and meat and potatoes. Of course, back then we ate a little bit more fat than we do now. By and large, I think diet has a lot to do with keeping a person in good physical condition. And sometimes, a little willpower helps to push the plate back.

"Of course, most of us, if we're healthy, can attribute a lot of that to our parents, who fed us well and took care of us when we were young. Today I consider myself in pretty good physical condition."

Fortunately, Joe also has a strong support system in both his doctor and his family. Lois, for instance, attends every race.

"She hasn't missed a race in 20 years," Joe said, proudly. "She does the timing. For most of the races we've gone to the last five years, there's another couple goes along to help. But before that, my wife and I would go alone. And if I have to change an engine or transmission, she knows which end of a wrench is the business end.

"Since Sports Car Club of America is a volunteer organization, it requires volunteer work, and my wife is the chief registrar for our local division. She even once went through racing driver's school! She decided she didn't want to be a race driver."

Even their son gets into the act. Joseph Hauser III also started racing after serving a stint in the Air Force.

"In fact, one year at the run-offs, about 1981, we ended first and second!" Joe said. "I was first."

Consequently, Joe thinks racing is the ultimate sport. It is, he says, one of the few sports where 70-year-olds can compete on a level track with 20-year-olds. Racing's message of fun and equality is one he preaches every chance he gets.

"I tell people, 'Get you a car and go racing!'" Joe said. "Anybody can go racing! Of course, since this organization is basically a not-for-profit deal with no prize money, a lot of people can't afford to go racing until they get their kids through college. I did, but it was by basically squeezing a little here and there until we had enough.

"I've also had guys 55–60 come up to me and say, 'Boy, I wish I could do that!' I say, 'Sure, why not?' I think the main thing a lot of people don't realize is that they don't lose technique or abilities—well, some people might—but people who are healthy mentally and physically, there's no reason they couldn't go racing when they're 60 and 70.

"There are a lot of people flying at ages 65–75, although I think race driving is a little more complex than piloting a light airplane. As far as danger goes, flying might be a little more dangerous. Because, while we do have an occasional fatality, there are good controls. All the cars have to pass safety inspections; the drivers have to pass physicals."

To prove his point, Joe, like 67-year-old actor/racer/chef Paul Newman, is a member of a Denver, Colorado-based organization called the Chevaliers. Membership is restricted to active, competitive car racers over the age of 50.

"I keep saying I'm going to quit one of these years," Joe said. "I'm getting lazy. I don't hate to lose as much as I used to! And so I don't really put as much effort into my car as I used to. And I've been doing it for so long.

"Still, I figure I've got a few more years, assuming I'm still in good physical and mental condition. I don't know why I wouldn't be—but at my age, who knows? But then, that's true of anybody.

"I don't think I've changed a lot since I started racing in the 1960s," Joe told *USA Today*. "Except I've gotten 30 years older."

And better.

Chapter 11

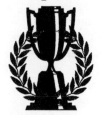

Pat Henninges

CARLTON, TEXAS—Pat Henninges is one tough cookie. At age 64, she continues to take a regular pounding on three southwestern barrel-racing circuits. She's been a top winner for the past several years, even though she often competes in the 45-and-over category.

Just *how* tough is Pat?

Consider this story from January 17, 1988, in Cleburne, Texas. The setting is a small arena at a nearby ranch. Pat has horses entered in both the $50 novice class and the $500 novice class.

Unlike most barrel-racing arenas, this particular arena has an unusual feature to it. Riders can't exit into adjoining pastures following a run unless a heavy wire gate is lifted first. Before her first run, Pat checked carefully to see that the gate was indeed open.

"I made my run and when I came out, I thought I had the pasture to go out into," she said. "But the sun was pretty bad and I couldn't see. And somebody had closed that gate into the pasture and I didn't see it. But the horse did. He made a quick 90-degree turn.

"Now, I'm glad he turned because he had sense enough not to try to run through a wire gate. But when he turned, I was expecting to go straight. I went off and I mean to tell you I *hit* on my shoulder!"

Pat was tossed nearly 10 feet from her horse, which continued to run around the arena. Shaken, Pat began feeling around in the dirt for her eyeglasses.

"A bunch of people ran up and they were all asking if I was needing help," she said. "I said, 'No, I need to get my horse.' That's the first thing you think about—your horse.

"Once I recovered my horse, somebody brought a cold rag and wrapped it around my head because I was bleeding. But I had won on that particular horse by one second. My husband was there and he said, 'I told you you was gonna get killed... blah, blah, blah.' I said, 'Bob, I've got to hurry. I've got the $500 novice class to get another horse in.' He shouted, 'You're not going back to ride in there!' I said, 'Yes, I am going to ride, too.' 'No, you're not.' 'Yes, I am.'

"Well, I got to ride and I won first in that $500 class, too! I did it the hard way!"

You can't tell Pat Henninges' story without telling about the horses in her life. And horses have been an integral part of her life since growing up on a ranch near Lampkin, Texas.

"When I was a little girl, I didn't have a horse at first, and I wanted a horse so bad that I had stick horses," she said. "I could *visualize* those horses as beautiful horses! When we moved to Lampkin and I went to school, I was so thrilled because Daddy got me a horse. Horses have always been my first love.

"Back in those days, we didn't have buses to ride to school, so we rode horses. As a kid, my big dream was to have a horse, and when I finally got one, I rode him every day, in cold or hot weather. We finally got us a little ol' school bus during my later grammar school years, but I always liked riding my horse better."

After graduating from high school, Pat left home and went to work for Western Union. It was the last time she was able to be involved with her beloved horses for nearly 40 years.

Along the way, she did find time to get married to Bob Henninges. Bob's goal was to be a pilot and work as an air traffic controller.

"What Bob wanted to do was anything to do with airplanes," Pat said. "From the time our daughter was young, he spent much of his time at the airport, so I went along. I'd kick those tires, too. Pretty soon I started taking flying lessons and I did get my pilot's license. Part of that was that I wanted to get into the air traffic controllers like Bob. But the other part was just to be with him."

In the following years, she worked first for the Civil Service, then at the veterans' hospital at Fort Hood, near Killeen, Texas. Eventually, she went to work for the Federal Aviation Administration in Fort Worth.

"I started out as a teletype operator because, back in those days, they didn't think much of women air traffic controllers," she said. "I kept trying to get in, and after overcoming several obstacles, I finally did get into air traffic school. I did what it took to make it."

Following her training period, Pat worked in both Mineral Wells and Fort Worth.

"We used to fly an awful lot when our daughter was in high school and college," Pat said. "Bob used to fly a Bonanza and I had a Cherokee. When I first started working in Mineral Wells, I'd occasionally fly to Mineral Wells to work! But I got rid of my airplane a long time ago, and I never really was that crazy about flying. My first love was horses."

So for Pat, there was only one thing on her mind when she retired from the FAA in August 1984.

"The first thing I did in August was buy a horse," she said. "I hadn't done any riding in all those years."

At first she only rode her horse with her daughter and grandchildren. But, in time, the naturally competitive Pat began to hear about "Play Days." Play Days are informal riding meets that are sponsored by different organizations and are peculiar to the West and Southwest. Each Play Day has eight different speed events, like barrel racing, straight barrel, pylons, or flags. Riders compete year-round for points towards a spot in the national finals.

Although Pat was 56 and the age category for women was 45 and over, she began entering Play Days events anyway.

"At first I was just walking and trotting my horse through the events, because the horse I had didn't know those events," she said. "We both started from scratch. Gradually, trotting became loping.

"I enjoyed it so much I got a horse that had been trained to complete in the Play Days and he taught me more at that first Play Day than I had learned up to that point! He was a real nice horse. That was my first taste of what it was like to really be competitive with a horse."

Unfortunately, Pat's horses were having trouble with colic. Finally, she took them to a veterinary college where she was told that the horses needed to be turned out more to free pasture.

"This was hard, living in a Fort Worth suburb," she said. "We had a ranch near Lampkin where we went on the weekends. My husband was still an air traffic controller then, so I moved down to the ranch with my horses. Later he retired and joined me.

"That's when I began doing more barrel racing and joined the West Texas Barrel Racing Association in 1986. I remember the secretary said when I joined, 'You're going to need a pretty good horse to compete in the 45 and over category.' From then on, I was the oldest contestant at every meet."

She also quickly became one of the most successful. In 1987, her first full year of competing in barrel racing, Pat finished fifth in the standings in the 45 and older category.

"In 1988, I got third place," she said. "In 1989, I finished first and got a saddle. And in 1990, I also finished first overall and got a saddle. In 1991, I got second place. So far in 1992, I've gone to fewer meets, but I hauled pretty good there for several years!

"I'm also a member of the Old Timers Rodeo Cowboy Association. In 1990, in the OTRCA, I finished third in the 50 and older category. In 1991, I got third in 50 and older, too.

"I also belong to the Lone Star Barrel Racing Association, where the category for women is 39 and over. In the final standings in 1991 I finished fifth there. I haven't been real high there—those girls are too tough for me. In 1992 I'm currently standing fourth, but I haven't hauled as much, so it may change. They only recognize the first five standings."

Despite the cash prizes, beautiful saddles, engraved belt buckles, and occasional media attention, Pat says the races have become a blur to her over the years. Only a few barrel races stand out in her mind.

"One I remember was when I bought a four-year-old horse in January 1987," she said. "That was the year it really rained a lot in January, so I didn't get on that horse much. But I took him to his first futurity in San Antonio in February. And I ran him and he made a real nice run. But he was a powerful horse and I'd never been on a horse that had that kind of speed.

"He was actually pretty sensible for a four-year-old. Usually when I would become unseated in the saddle, he would get back under me and he would try to wait on me at the barrel. Anyway, on the second run, I knew I had to hold him back."

The wet winter meant that Pat didn't ride competitively again until a March race in Mineral Wells. This was one of the premier barrel racing events of the season and many of the sport's top riders had entered.

"So here I was, an old lady with all of these young riders I'd read about in *Quarterhorse News*—so I'm scared to death," Pat said. "On his first run, my horse made a real nice, respectable run. But these kids—like Martha Wright—were just doing a lot better than I was. I should have been happy with my run. But I thought, 'Boy, I've got to show them in my second run.' So I asked that horse to really run.

"But what happened was my most embarrassing moment, because that horse *did* run to that first barrel and when I kicked him at the barrel, he got on his front end. Well, that almost threw me off. I was trying to climb back on while I was turning the horse at the same time around the first barrel—and all the while he's trying to come under to keep me from falling off! He was doing everything he was supposed to do."

Just then the animal veered towards the high fence that surrounded the arena. Pat, who was hanging on to the horse's powerful neck for dear life, decided she'd make a grab for the fence.

"And I thought, 'Boy, I'm going to be in a bind here!'" she recalled. "So I just turned him loose and I grabbed the top rail of the fence with one arm. My left hand grabbed that top rail—but I missed it with my right! Of course, my horse kept running. So my body got a pretty good jolt.

"I just kind of set myself down on the ground—although my shoulder was jolted pretty good in front of all of these people.

"*Embarrassed*—I was so embarrassed I didn't know what to do. That horse ran out and my right boot was still in the saddle because I'd rubber-banded my feet in the saddle. I always wore my boots real loose—thank goodness—or I'd have still been in there, too! My foot came out of the boot and the boot was still in the saddle. People came running up and said, 'Boy, that ol' boot is still just a kickin' that horse!'"

Sitting in the dirt and mud in Mineral Wells, Pat got to meet firsthand many of her heroes of barrel racing. A number of them vaulted over the fence and ran to her side the moment she hit the ground.

"I met all of those famous people after making a mess like that," she said. "I'll tell you, I met more people after that incident than at any other time. They came out into that arena and talked to me. They said things like, 'Are you all right?' 'Now, don't you quit barrel racing, we want you to keep on barrel racing.'

"Then they began telling me incidents that had happened to them, too! I guess everybody that's ever ridden a horse has had incidents. I've just probably had more than most people. I was pretty sore and I missed the next race the next month, but that was about all."

Barrel racing is a strenuous, sometimes dangerous sport. Riding a thousand-pound horse, running in a controlled gallop, and weaving between a number of closely set barrels requires both upper- and lower-body strength, balance, and endurance. Pat augments her regular practice rides—which invariably leave most riders and mounts wet with sweat—with a regular walking routine.

"But I don't really do a lot of additional exercise," she said. "I've always been a limber person. Before I run, a lot of times at the rodeos I get off to myself somewhere and touch my toes 10 times. I don't force it, because the first time I don't get very far, but then I get a little further. Even when I was a kid I couldn't touch my toes. But now at age 64, I've gotten to where, after so many bends, I can touch them."

She has also changed her diet in recent years, partly to keep her weight down and partly because she was found to have cholesterol levels that were too high.

"I don't have a doctor," she admits. "Neither my husband nor I really do. I've gone up there to Stephenville to a lady doctor for a physical and she kind of laughed at me when she found out I was a barrel racer. I don't really have time. I schedule an appointment when something comes up. I'm not a doctor person."

As Pat has continued barrel racing, she said her husband's interest in the sport has waned:

"He says, 'If you've seen one barrel race, you've seen them all. Mother, you're wearing me out, the horses, and the dog.' He wants me to cut back a little. He hardly ever goes now; it's a big deal when he goes. When we first started out, he was real good to go, but I guess I burned him out.

"Of course, the first years of our marriage were spent doing what *he* wanted to do. Here in the last part, I want to do what *I* want to do.

"It was always a dream of mine to have horses. So since I've retired, I've had horses. And I've got a place to keep 'em. Horses are my life right now—I've got five horses. Now it's *my* turn! I don't know what Bob thinks about it being my turn. He's pretty nice about it, except he says, 'You can't ever tell what those things are going to do.'"

There is, of course, a downside to owning horses, particularly ones that compete regularly in any rodeo event.

"Horses are prone to injuries and illnesses," she said. "You're always busy with horses because there's always something wrong. You keep the vets in business.

"I'll tell you what: There are a lot of peaks and valleys in this business. You'll be doing really good, then you'll get to be doing really terrible and you think, 'Gosh, I'm never going to win another barrel race!' And you think about selling your horse."

Pat says that most riders have periods of doubting their ability. They become depressed about a showing or an animal— or even the amount of time it takes to compete regularly. She says it is common among rodeo participants.

"I don't know that you'd say I'm optimistic," she said. "I have to make myself. I have to talk to myself because I get kind of down sometimes if I'm having horse problems or some horse is hurt. You know, you go to these vets and spend your money and you get a really good horse and find out later it has something wrong with it. Or if I do really bad in a race, I get down sometimes.

"Then I tell myself that that run is history and it really doesn't make any difference—it's the next run that counts. That's how I try to keep myself built up.

"One time when I got down, my daughter taped a barrel race off the TV. I was really depressed over my barrel racing and all back then. In the tape, though, this famous rider's horse went down on his front end and the rider ended up on his neck. It's terrible, but it made me feel better to know that even the champions have bad days. I felt good and started over again."

Unlike many sports, women's barrel racing has yet to develop a true "masters" classification. Pat sometimes competes against women who are nearly 25 years her junior. In fact, she's done it so long, she says she's used to it by now.

"One thing about competing with younger people is that it doesn't put as much pressure on you as when you compete with older people," she said. "So what if they beat you? I don't mind competing with them, but I could do with a 60-and-over class myself.

"Now, the OPRC rodeos are for 50 and over. The women at 50 seem pretty young when you're my age. A lot of those older women who do compete are good. A lot of them used to be on the circuit. They used to rodeo a long time ago, and I never did rodeo. So all of them are pretty tough and they've got some pretty tough horses. Plus, they had all of those years to rodeo that I now wish that I had had.

"But just because you missed it the first time around, doesn't mean you're too old."

Pat actively encourages young and old alike to give barrel racing a try. At times, she almost sounds like an evangelist when she touts the sport's merits. Then again, it's hard to argue with results. Most people would want to be as tough and vigorous as Pat is today at 64.

"A lot of times these girls think they're old when they're 30!" she said. "They'll want to start barrel racing or something and I'll encourage them and tell them to go ahead. I'll say, 'Hey, I didn't start until I was in my 50s. So you go ahead and do it. Don't be shy.'

"I tell them to start at any Play Day, get you a horse, and walk or trot your way through it. And gradually go from there.

"I've got a girl right now that I'm encouraging a lot. I told her she had the perfect horse—which she has for sale. I told her I wished I had that horse. I said, 'Why don't you start riding it?'—because she used to ride when she was young. She said, 'I'm going to start one of these days.'

"I said, 'Do it now because *that* is the perfect horse. It just doesn't have any holes, and it's hard to find a horse that doesn't have any holes in it.' She thinks she's going to start and I'm hoping she does."

Still, Pat is modest to a fault ("I don't think I inspire anybody."), despite her success on the circuit.

"I've had a lot of people come up to me and say nice things," she grudgingly admits, "but I'm sure others are thinking, 'Who is that crazy old lady out there?'"

Even today, when complimented after an especially fine showing at a tough San Antonio barrel race, she quickly turns the conversation elsewhere. She gives the credit to her husband, her daughter, her grandchildren, her horses (Mr. Shiney Chick, Scat's Sparkle, Scooter, and Sorrelly), *everybody* but her dog Pretzel.

"Somebody who has been helpful to me is Martha Josey," Pat said. "I've been to three of her barrel racing clinics. At the first one I went to, the kids were still interested in barrel racing and we were a three-generation family there: me, my daughter, and both of her children! Ed Wright has also been real helpful to me, especially with my horses. He's really a good trainer. And a lot of these kids on the circuit helped me a lot, people like Larry Stevens. When you're riding, there's always somebody you can go to.

"If I have a problem with a horse, I realize I've got a problem, and I take it to someone who can get on the horse and look it over so I can handle it. There's something to keeping a horse tuned. I don't like horses that don't work. I want a horse that's patterned, that does a good job. If I start having a problem with one, usually I try to get some help to figure out if it is me or the horse!"

With Pat's track record, bet that it is the horse that's having trouble.

The smart money's always on Pat Henninges. Win, place, or show.

Chapter 12

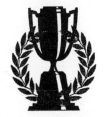

Jim Law

CHARLOTTE, NORTH CAROLINA—One of the highlights of the 1991 Senior Games in Syracuse was the 400-meter dash in the 65–69 age bracket. The two top contenders, Jim Law of Charlotte, North Carolina, and Willie Blackmon of Columbus, Ohio, lined up nervously at the starting gate. The 400 is a crowd favorite, but the participants aren't particularly fond of it.

"It's a very grueling race," Jim said later. "I'm convinced that, of the sprints, it is the Mother of Masochism. I don't know why we do that stuff, but we do."

On this day, Jim did it again. Both Jim and Willie got tremendous jumps at the gun and flew around the track, neither giving an inch. The entire crowd was roaring as one, urging the two men on. Until that race, the 60-second barrier had never been broken in the 400 meters in the 65-and-up age bracket.

"But in the finals that day, both of us broke not just 60 seconds, but 59 seconds," Jim said. "Though I hit the finish line first, Willie really had the better performance because he was a year older than I was.

"Still, I was just very excited to have the two of us with our Medicare cards coming in under 59 seconds!"

That feat was remarkable enough in itself. But earlier in the meet, Jim Law had broken the age bracket records in both the 100- and 200-meter dashes as well!

Since returning to competition in 1986 after a 40-year lay-off, Jim has won a wall full of gold and silver medals for the various sprints and relays, as well as five gold and seven silver medals in international competition.

Oh, and one other thing. Jim won the 100-, 200-, and 400-meter dashes in the 1989 Senior Games in St. Louis, as well—competing in the 60–64 age bracket.

Jim was born in Baltimore in 1926. His father, also Jim Law, had been a marvelous athlete in his day at Lincoln University in Pennsylvania. Eighteen years later, Jim Jr. attended the same school.

"I did not grow up in his household, so there was not the environmental stuff going on, but I suspect some genetic things were going on," Jim said. "It was when I started doing athletics in college that I got the name 'Jim'. I wasn't even sure I knew I was a 'Jim' until that time, because I had been called by my middle name, Roland. But people who knew my father as an athlete started referring to me as 'Young Jim.' That's where Jim Law came about, really because of my father's prowess, and my following him."

At Lincoln, Jim participated in both basketball and track, and earned some notoriety for ability on the cinders.

In 1939, Jim took a position at Johnson C. Smith University, a small liberal arts college in Charlotte, North Carolina.

"I came here in 1939 in order to get one year's experience in teaching," Jim said. "My wife tells me that that establishes clearly that there is such a thing as a slow learner, because I've been here ever since—44 years—except for a few leaves of absence where I've gone to study or to teach somewhere else.

"My discipline is psychology—experimental psychology, as I hasten to tell some folks."

A few years ago, the administration offered Jim the post of vice-president of academic affairs.

"There is a comic who says he has a microwave fireplace, and that enables him to spend an entire evening in front of the fireplace in eight minutes," Jim said. "I was like that. I was a fast-food junkie, getting things in a hurry so I could get back to work. I was eating the wrong kinds of things. I was dashing about every hour.

"Post-college, I did nothing athletically for a while. I was pretty fit in high school and in college. But then I did what happens in this country—I sat down for 40 years."

It was while he was an administrator at Johnson C. Smith that he read a short article in the Charlotte newspaper that piqued his interest.

"In 1985, I saw this ad about some Senior Games here," he said. "My eyes fell on table tennis, which is one of my enthusiasms. I entered and I won! A couple of months later, I went on to the state competition and I won there.

"But more important than me winning table tennis is that I

noticed people my age were running! I had no idea that people my age were doing that running thing!"

It wasn't long before Jim was doing "that running thing" himself, getting into shape—and loving it.

Something else happened. Jim realized that he didn't like working in administration.

"I think, in part, that's because I got into running while I was in that position," he said. "I think I elected, because of that association with track, to go back to teaching where I belong. It was an interesting experience and I got some things accomplished and others I didn't get accomplished. But I tell you, I belong in the classroom. Senior Games and athletics helped me appreciate that."

So Jim ran for the first time the following year, 1986, and won the local meet.

"Before getting ready to compete in running, I decided to go to the doctor," Jim said. "That's backwards, of course. You should go to the doctor first, but that wasn't my style.

"Once I got to him, the doctor put my running on hold because he thought he detected some blockages here and there and wanted to do further tests. It turned out that the blockages he suspected were not confirmed—and I'm grateful for that— but he did find a very serious cholesterol problem."

Serious, indeed! Jim's first cholesterol reading was a whopping 322.

"The doctor talked about the need for shifting my diet and for doing some regular exercise," Jim said. "I took him seriously. But I did him one better. I started taking cooking lessons in macrobiotics. I did that for a while, and it took six or seven months for my cholesterol reading to fall from 322 to 188. But I've brought it down further, and the most recent reading I've had is 127.

"I think it was a combination of nutrition and exercise. I went mainly to whole grains and vegetables and cut down tremendously on the kinds of red meat I would eat. I'm not a fanatic who won't eat anything like that, but I went mostly to fish and fowl. And now I find that we have many, many meals per week without any meat at all. And it's not like I decided that this is what I was going to do, but it evolved that way and I'm grateful for it.

"Now what I eat takes a long time to prepare, and it takes me longer to eat it. And I think that is beneficial. It is a different way of living, it's not a 'microwave' way of living.

"And that leaves me very high on Senior Games because I'm not sure I'd be alive today had I not gotten involved with Senior Games and undergone the interventions that followed."

Armed with a new lifestyle and his old job back, Jim began regular training in 1987. As he had done in college, he chose to specialize in the 100-, 200- and 400-meter sprints.

In 1989, Jim qualified for the Senior Games in St. Louis in all three events.

"And I had a grand time," he said. "I won my three events— the 100-, 200-, 400-meters—and set Senior Games records in the 60–64 age group.

"In 1991, I repeated that. I won them again, but by then I was in the 65–69 age bracket and once again set records for that age group.

"I'm going to Baton Rouge in '93, but it is going to be tougher because I'll be older. Two years ago I was a snot-nosed 65. But it won't be as bad as it was in my first one. I'll be 67 and there will be two more years in my age group ahead of me, so it should be easier than the first one, but not as easy as the second one. This is, of course, just sheer speculation on my part!"

On the other hand, Jim's track record in the past has been pretty good on such things.

There have been, of course, many other races between 1987 and today. Jim professes to remembering few details about most of them. And the few races he does remember generally aren't the victories.

"I was in TAC (The Athletic Congress) nationals in Indianapolis in the 400 meters when I was 64," he recalled. "I had lane 5, and the world record holder in the 60-64 age bracket, Jack Greenwood, was in lane 6 or 7. He was outside of me.

"Because Jack was on the outside, I kept my eye on him the whole way. Things were going ever so well when, lo and behold as we hit the final turn, a couple of those young guys—61 or so—started streaking by me in the turn. We were going too slowly. I didn't know that Jack Greenwood was not in fine fettle physically that day; I had no idea. Anyway, I had to start kicking up my gears and I ultimately won it by a nip.

"It was a very fine lesson for me: run your game, stop looking at other people. That was my mistake, and that has stuck with me ever since."

But if you work to pin him down, Jim will admit an unabashed preference for the relays. And, as before, his international record is almost unblemished as a member of both the 4 x 100- and 4 x 400-meter relay teams.

"I love relays," he said. "There is something about them. Perhaps being part of a team makes it special. One of my favorite races was in 1989 in Eugene, Oregon,—called by many the track capital of the country, some say the track capital of the world—and they do have a marvelous enthusiasm for track. I was on both the 4 x 1 and 4 x 4 relays and we set records for our age group that day.

"But the most memorable was in the World Veterans Championships in Finland in 1991. I went to Finland sick and injured. I was in bad shape. And that was to have been my year. I had just turned 65, I was the new kid on the block, and I'd run pretty well in the nationals, where I'd set world records in the 400-meter dash for my age group.

"But I hurt myself at the nationals; I pulled a hamstring in the 100 and had to sort of hobble in the 100 and 200, although I did finish second in both of those.

"On top of that, I had a virus and I had just left from the Senior Olympics. There was only one day between the Senior Olympics and the Nationals. It was just too much strain for me to do and I ended up with a virus. But my doctor said I should go, so I went. The physical therapist in Finland kept me running—ultrasound and Finnish fingers!"

Still, Jim's performances were below his standard in all three events. Fortunately, the final day of the World Veterans Championships were devoted strictly to the relays.

"There was some healing by then, and there was the added motivation of doing it as a team," he said. "In the 4 x 4, we picked the folks who do best in the open 400. We had two fellows who hadn't made the finals in the 400, but we didn't have that many people there to chose from, so they ran the first two legs. We got the baton in third place, but we ended up winning the whole thing. I was especially pleased for those two fellows because neither had ever won a gold medal in a world competition. We had a grand time! That was probably the best time I remember in a race because we were able to pull that one out and get the gold for America. So I enjoy relays especially."

To get to that level of competition, much less win multiple gold and silver medals, Jim Law is obviously blessed with blazing speed and—particularly in the 400 meters—iron-willed endurance. That kind of combination can only come through an almost fanatical devotion to the most rigorous training routine devised by man, right?

Well, sort of.

"I wish I could tell you that my exercise regimen was terribly systematic," Jim said, almost apologetically. "There is a lot of jazz in my routine—a lot of improvisation from day to day. But one thing I decided early, and I continue to follow it now: I don't run every day. I run about three times a week. And I do this because it seems to me that the older you get, the more time your body needs to recover from what things have been visited upon it.

"One of the things I've done with my colleagues is try to keep them from overtraining, doing too much. I think I've succeeded with one or two in getting them to pull back because we're especially susceptible when we get older. Less is more. I've held to that—not training too much."

The only time Jim runs on consecutive days is at major, multi-day track meets.

"I run sprints mostly in my workouts," he said. "I don't do the long stuff because I'm doing the short, fast stuff. That's what I practice at. Not that I'm out doing it all the time. I'm working on technique and this, that, and the other. I feel bad when I don't get those three days in."

Jim must drive for an hour each day to run on a standard public track. Otherwise, he runs on area soccer fields, which generally have the most level surfaces.

"When I get in those days, I feel good," Jim said. "I'm sure that it is traceable to the endorphines. I once thought that they were limited to distance runners. But not so. I'm a sprinter, and I get the same kind of euphoria from doing that stuff three times a week that cyclists and distance runners get. It is really an exercise high that is associated with the release of endorphines. That's important, that keeps me going.

"I'm out there anywhere from 30 minutes to one and a half hours, depending on what needs to be done and how I feel."

Despite the vagaries of the conditions—and bad weather can curtail Jim's outdoor workouts—he says that there has been an unexpected benefit from running on the soccer fields. He says he's gotten re-acquainted with Mother Nature—for the first time in 40 years.

"I'd spent most of my years looking at glass and concrete and asphalt," he said, "but once again I can now appreciate grass and foliage and rabbits and birds. In my town, there are a couple of Canadian geese that stay here year round, and every so often they plop down on the soccer field while I'm running and I undergo a fit of joy.

"One of the great benefits that's come to me from getting re-involved in track is to appreciate nature again. We don't do as much of that as we need, I'm sure."

On his "off" days, Jim has a more organized schedule of cross-training activities.

"One son left some weights at home, which I use from time to time—not with great joy, but I use them because while most people think of running as only a leg activity, there is also a need for upper-body strength," he said. "So I do the weights. We've also got some other kinds of things around here: a stepper, a rower, and a cross-county ski machine.

"The other thing I use is water. I'm off to the pool every so often. I've got one of these things where you can run in the water. I use it, especially if I'm injured. Water is naturally therapeutic in the first place and it has a resistance that will keep you in shape while avoiding the impact that running on a hard surface would involve.

"I think cross-training is important because it gives you some variety and because you keep your muscles in balance. If you do the same thing all the time, your front stuff is going to get stronger than your back stuff. So cross-training is a definite part of what I do for exercise."

Jim says, knowing what he knows now, that he'd be doing all of this running and cross-training even if he weren't competing in track on an international level.

"There is all kinds of evidence for seniors that regular activities benefit your everything: muscles, bones, cholesterol, blood pressure, all of that stuff," he said. "And they are not just physical gains either. You're better off emotionally, physically—even tranquility is more likely to be yours if you do all of that.

"All of us need to do this thing. Life is movement; we've got to get ourselves into moving pretty regularly—prudently, though—so that we can help ourselves."

Since his first scary brush with a doctor, Jim said he's made medical checkups a regular part of his routine. To date, all of his doctors have been supportive of his increased activity level. Some, in fact, even use him as an example of what *can* be done.

"Nutrition and exercise—and there are other things as well—

these are the things that changed me around," said Jim.

A lifestyle change of that magnitude couldn't have gone unnoticed in his own household, of course. Both of his sons, ages 30 and 34, are physically active. But the real story is his wife, Aurelia.

"Aurelia has no athletic history at all," Jim said, "but she started running with me when I started running in '86. And she did well. She came in second in the 100. And since that time, she's added the 200 meters. She stayed off it for a couple years because she had some blood pressure problems, but she came back this year and won both the 100 and the 200 meters in her age group at the state level. So Aurelia has now qualified to go to Baton Rouge, too!

"When I lecture, I use her as an example to say, 'You can come at it even if you have no history of exercise at all. You can start, even late in life, and even achieve some competence— but you will definitely feel better and look better physically by doing such a program.' My own case illustrates that if you started way back there and used to do it—but didn't do it for a while—it is possible to come back! Even though it may be hard, it is possible."

Jim is currently on a one-year leave-of-absence from teaching to take part in a cross-country lecture tour on the benefits of— what else?—exercise and nutrition. He says he's been addressing both his fellow "elderlies" and young people along the eight-city circuit.

"My advice for young people who want to stay fit in their 60s is to stay in condition," he said. "If they're already there— stay there!

"So many young athletes end up doing nothing once they finish school. One thing we can do organizationally is to set it up so there are opportunities for them to engage in activities once they leave school. The TAC, which starts at age 30 for what is called the sub-masters, should be even lower—25, maybe even 20, so that there is no gap between what happens in school and when they can enter masters' events.

"My encouragement to young folk is to stay active. I do my best to keep them active and to talk to them about the need for that. What I say to them is that they will miss out on much of the exhilaration of life if they're going to become sedentary. They're just missing so much life by not being active. That's the kind of point I've been trying to make with them. I haven't been turned down lately, not that I've got everybody doing everything. That's my pitch to the young folk: life is movement."

Jim says that even those sports once thought to be the exclusive domain of the young are still open to people who remain active all their lives.

"We've got 3 on 3 basketball in the Senior Games for ages 65 and up," he said. "Jack McCloskey, who is the general manager of the Detroit Pistons, won it last year. I've been threatening him to gather unto myself a team to challenge him in Baton Rouge. They've also added softball and volleyball and these team things are going on in a competitive way, but among oldsters. You don't have to get rid of a particular sport. I think that young folk just need to be turned on to the importance of continuing active lifestyles."

But there may be much more to it than just the fitness aspects. There must be something stronger still that would compel otherwise normal seniors into a serious training regimen when many of their friends are at home in their rocking chairs.

Jim says there is: the people.

"The association with the people I meet in the events is somehow spiritual," he said. "I have never seen such sharing and caring as among senior athletes. They will give tips to one another just before they race each other. They will share any information. All of that, I think, is kind of special.

"I have been involved in my community in volunteerism, so I'm very high on helping other folks. It gives me optimism for humankind to see folks helping one another. And how nice it was to learn that one can get endorphines when you help other people! It's the same as runner's high, but you only get it from a face-to-face situation, not by just writing a check. How nice it is to be rewarded for doing something we ought to be doing anyhow."

Another positive side effect of working out and competing is that optimism Jim mentioned. He says he's never met a senior competitor yet who wasn't optimistic, either about his ability or his health.

"Optimism is a tremendously important ingredient anywhere along the way, but especially the older you get," Jim said.

"Another element of that is that we are more likely to see our difficulties as traceable to a particular disease, disorder or injury, rather than the aging process itself. As long as you think it is the aging process itself, you are in trouble. People give up under those circumstances.

"I plan to run forever. I like forever. I have no plans to give it up unless I go to something else. I'd like to try tennis for a while, but I don't think I'll give up running, whatever happens."

Not surprisingly, optimistic, positive people look to the future. Jim recently signed up for a class in conversational Japanese in preparation for his October 1993 trip to Japan for the World Veterans Championships there. Unfortunately, the class was later cancelled because of insufficient registrations.

"One *needs* to be active," he said. "Like they say, if you don't use it, you'll lose it—and that's true of physical things and mental things as well. I do look forward to the future. I have short-term goals.

"For instance, there are several of us right now who are trying to see how we'll get through 1993's three key events in track and field: we've got our National Senior Games, which are held every other year; we've got our national annual TAC event; *and* we've got the World Veterans Championships in Japan, also held every other year. Those things all take place between June and October and some of us are in despair at trying to peak three different times! Me, I'll deal with the peaking when the time comes!"

One interesting sideline of the Jim Law story is how completely he has dominated his events in recent years. He is even considering adding additional events, like the discus, long jump, and hurdles—a thought that unnerves more than a few of the athletes in those events. But Jim says domination has never interested him.

"One of the things that happens in regard to this stuff is that you get more creative in your goal setting as you get more mature," he said. "It may be nice to win, there may be something special about that, I guess. But I'm in for the participation much more than the winning.

"What I'm looking for—and what I try to get others to look for—is continued growth. Now, sometimes that means you want to do better than you have recently done—PRs (personal records) are the things you look at within particular age groups.

"We can be creative in our goal setting, we can try to find victory in unexpected places. It is not my goal to dominate all the time—heavens no! It is to win and run well. Winning is not the largest thing for me.

"There also may be a time when you're looking at deteriorating less than expected! That's a goal too, and that can work for you. George Sheehan talks about *not* competing against the folks who are in front of you, but competing against the little guy inside of you who wants to quit. He who finishes the race has won!"

Chapter 13

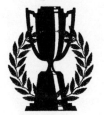

"Tuffy" Roy Overturf

ODESSA, TEXAS—Roy Houston "Tuffy" Overturf is as tough as West Texas tank water. He's a raunchy little cowboy, a tough, sinewy 78-year-old, and a stiff-walking, slow-talking, calf-roping machine. And he's got a voice as raspy as fingernails on a metal file. Or maybe it's just rusty because he doesn't use it much. Tuffy Overturf is one of the last of the old-time cowboys. Polite, laconic, and soft-spoken—when he speaks at all.

But Tuffy Overturf is all business in the rodeo arena. He comes darting out of the chute low, a second rope clenched tightly in his mouth. His equally wiry little pony, Dude, leans ahead momentarily and Tuffy explodes forward, sending his rope just in front of the frantic calf.

The animal spins to a stop and is yanked roughly to the dirt floor. Tuffy darts to the calf's side, and ties the rope in a knot around its spindly legs in a series of windmilling arm motions.

This time, however, the calf squeals and lashes out while Tuffy attempts to complete the tie-down. When he finally throws his arms in the air to signal he is finished, 16 seconds have elapsed. Tuffy disgustedly remounts Dude and trots slowly back to the starting gate. The other cowboys file by: "Tough luck, Tuffy." "You'll get him next time, podnuh."

And he did, too. Through the summer of 1992, Tuffy Overturf was taking home more than his share of the prize money at the National Old Timers Calf Roping Association's weekly rodeos across Texas. Along the way, he was beating men, 10, 15—sometimes even 20—years younger.

The Tuffy Overturf story began in 1914 in Big Spring, about 60 dusty miles from Odessa in West Texas. His stepfather was a carpenter, and Tuffy went to work building oil-storage tanks in

1937 for Mapp Tank Co. It was at Mapp that "Roy Houston" was forever transformed into "Tuffy."

"There was an old gentleman working there named E. N. Maples," Tuffy drawled. He started calling me 'Overtuff' instead of 'Overturf.' That turned into 'Overtuffy,' and eventually 'Tuffy' got to be my name. It kinda stuck."

Incidentally, Tuffy remained at Mapp until he retired in 1981.

"I started riding when I was a kid," Tuffy recalled. "I worked for the famous Cauble Ranch near Big Spring and that's where I got the idea of roping. The owner's son roped and I was out there helping him. I always liked horses; I've always messed with horses. I've played golf and this, that, and the other—but I discovered that I'd always rather rope."

Although Tuffy quickly became adept at the intricate sport, he never roped professionally. Sometimes he'd rope for fun and at amateur shows on weekends. And in the days following his reluctant retirement, he only occasionally tried his hand at the sport.

"For four or five years after my retirement," Tuffy said, "my son, Shirl, tried to get me to go to some of the senior roping rodeos, but I wouldn't go, see. I was doing something else, although I don't know just what now. I was still working a lot. Finally, I decided I'd start coming. Since I've retired, that's all I've got to do."

Tuffy soon joined the National Old Timers Calf Roping Association. The group organizes monthly ropings and awards points based on performance. At the end of the riding year, cash prizes, belt buckles, and saddles are awarded to the top calf ropers in each age group.

The money for the prizes comes from an entry fee collected from each roper for each individual event—generally about $50. The entry fees also cover the costs of livestock, transportation, arena rental, and association salaries.

"There's also an Old Timers Rodeo Association of South Texas," Tuffy said. "Bill Dunlap goes to all of them. I went to them for a year or two, but they got to be so far away that I couldn't go. I didn't have nobody to go with and my wife, she give out on me pretty quick! But I got another old boy who don't live far from me near Odessa who just turned 71 and we can start going together.

"You couldn't make a living at it. But it helps."

Not that Tuffy and his prized horse Dude do all that badly.

"I don't know how many ropings I've won over the years," Tuffy said. "Several, I'd say. I was Champion Calf Roper over in Abilene in 1991 in the 71-and-older age group. But I also compete in the 65-and-over age group. I won that age group up in Abilene in July 1992, and I've placed in that category five–six times since I started this."

Of course, there is more to calf roping than belt buckles and saddles.

"When I leave that chute, all I'm thinking about is ropin' that sonuvagun, getting to him, and tyin' him down," Tuffy said, "and beatin' them other guys, beatin' them old codgers! Everything is focused on that task. You can holler and yell and everything else, I don't even hear you.

"The other thing is, in this Old Timers circuit, everybody knows everybody, and everybody helps one another all the time: getting the calves out, keeping the horses straight in the chute so you can get out on them, that stuff. They all work together; they're a good bunch of men."

That camaraderie is no small part of the attraction for the old cowboys.

"The friends, the visits, sure is—if it wasn't for that, I wouldn't go, probably."

Despite the sometimes dangerous nature of the sport, Tuff said none of his major injuries through the years have come from calf roping.

Not that it would matter if they had.

"My doctors don't tell me *not* to rope," he said. "They know I do it and they know I'll do it anyway.

"And my family has been real supportive. I've got two more generations roping. I've got a son who ropes all the time and a grandson who is roping in the college ranks—and that's pretty tough."

Stiffness in his knees limits Tuffy's regular exercise routine— except for roping, of course.

"My exercise is that I rope three–four times a week at home," he said. "I've got my own arena and my own calves and some good horses. But I get a lot of exercise calf roping. This is about as good an exercise as you can get.

"I'm not in any better shape than I was when I first retired because of the roping, but I'm still in good shape—considering my age. Seventy-eight is getting on up there.

"I've always tried to stay in shape. I'll go in the house and sit on the couch and watch TV for an hour or two and I'll get to hurtin' all over and I've got to get up and get to movin' all around. I've got arthritis in my hands. I'd attribute my shape to working all my life, and staying active, and doing stuff."

That, incidentally, is the advice he gives to both young and old when they ask how they can still be roping at age 78.

"Just stay active, just stay active, and just keep on going and doing," he said. "You've *got* to have exercise, you've *got* to have that. Riding my horses and roping is exercise. This is good exercise. You can't beat it, I don't guess.

"And for somebody nearing retirement age, I tell them just to have at it, but don't overdo it at first. Because you can overdo it, you know. You can get too hot out there roping or something."

With Tuffy Overturf, the discussion always seems to turn back to calf roping. What *is* the attraction of roping?

"I just like it, I guess," he said. "I don't know, it just appealed to me better. You've got to have a good horse, he's got to work, y'all got to work together or it's no good.

"I'm going to ride as long as I feel like it. It's fun every day that I. I rope at home all of the time. I feel that, as long as the Man Upstairs will let me do this, I'll do it."

Still, getting Tuffy to talk about himself is like pulling teeth with a worn set of pliers. But ask Tuffy about his favorite subject—horses—and suddenly he's a garrulous cowboy philosopher, waxing poetic on the virtues of the noble beast:

"A man and a good horse can think together. I had a little bay horse I roped on for nine years, and that rascal could go up and down that arena! And if a calf wouldn't veer off to the right, he'd move to make the calf go a little to the right—and that's when I'd rope him! We clicked together pretty good.

"But not every horse. Just some horses. You can train a horse to do anything you want them to do. But there's some that's better than others. It don't take long to tell: maybe three weeks or a month. You can tell pretty quick. Other cowboys can tell by watching the way he acts, what he does."

Not surprisingly, Tuffy continues to train horses, both for himself and for friends.

"I let my grandson ride 'em, but I watch him and see what he does, and tell him what he does that's right," Tuffy said. "Of course, he's 23 years old, so he's roped a few calves in his life. A horse is about 90 percent of a successful roper. Of course, you've got to be able to use him."

But if the horse is 90 percent of calf roping, what does that leave the roper?

"You've got to do the same thing every time," Tuffy mused. "You put your horse in the same place and do the same thing or he won't catch on to what you're trying to do. It ain't no cinch any way you want to take it.

"What makes a good roper is practice. Ropin' all the time and going. It's work, ain't no two ways about it."

On this particular day at the rodeo, Tuffy is riding Dude, a tough little pony that prances nervously around the arena.

"There's no telling what I could get for that little horse," Tuffy said with a nod towards Dude. "Everywhere I go, there's somebody tryin' to buy him. He's a dandy, he's a dandy. He's little, but he has such a big heart. And run? You see how he can run? That little sonuvagun can fly. He's the smallest little horse I've had, but Dude's a tough one. He's good.

"I call him 'Dude' 'cause he's so jumpy. I bought him for my grandson. I paid two calves for him and I was going to train him for my grandson, but turned out he's so good, I said, 'Wait a minute! That grandson don't need this horse. I do!' He don't care too much about roping right now anyway.

"One boy walked up to me at a roping about a year ago and said, 'Tuffy, what's it going to take to buy that horse?' I said, 'He's not for sale.' As long as I'm gonna ride, I might as well ride him."

On this particular summer day, Tuffy Overturf finishes tied for third place in the over-71 age group. Afterwards, he begins to brush down Dude for the long haul back to Odessa.

One last question: Have you ever had a perfect ride?

"Years ago," he says, "I'd tie 'em in 9 or 10 seconds—I mean, that was *30* years ago!" he said solemnly. "Today, about 12–13 is average, up to 16–17 seconds.

"Still, you do that and Son, you're going to place."

For the moment, the world holds nothing more alluring, no grander inducement than that, to Tuffy Overturf.

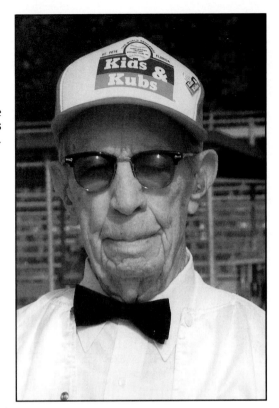

George A. Bakewell is not only the starting catcher for Kids & Kubs, he's the poet laureate as well.

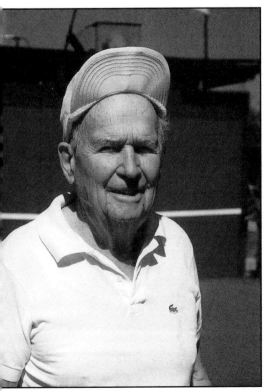

Ken Beer has played tennis throughout Asia and North America.

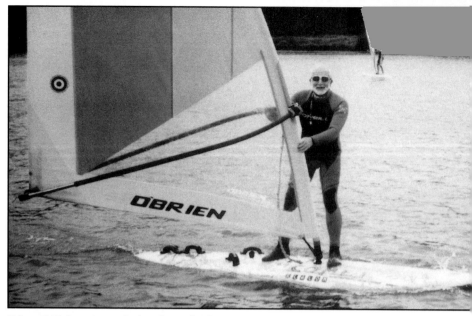

Edward Bishop is a windsurfing whiz!

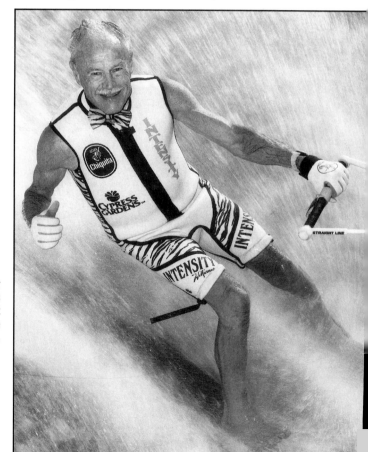

George Blair
goes bananas
over barefoot
skiing and the
color yellow.

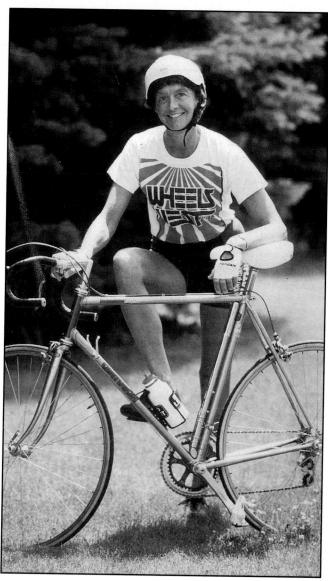

Sister Madonna Buder considers each Ironman Triathlon a prayer to God.

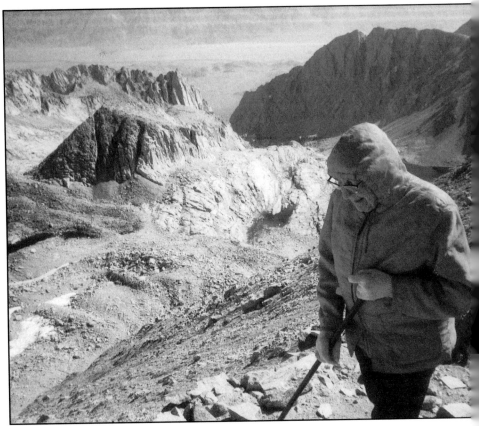

Hulda Crooks' lifelong love affair with mountain-climbing has taken her to the tops of some of the tallest mountains in California.

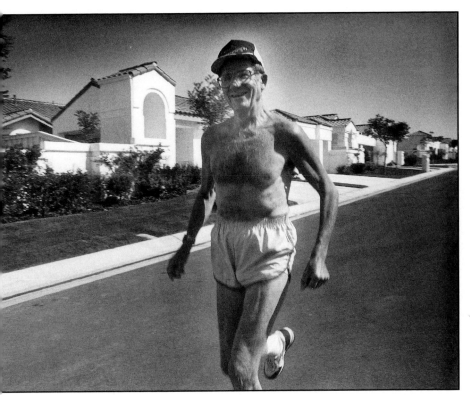

orton Davey alternates between Ironman Triathlons and full marathons.

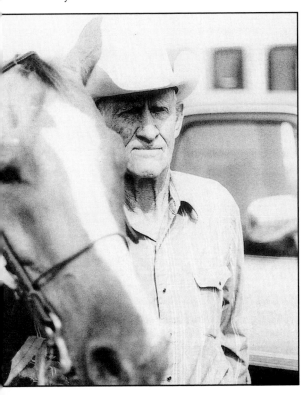

Bill Dunlap is one of the National Old Timers Calf Roping Association's oldest—and toughest—cowboys.

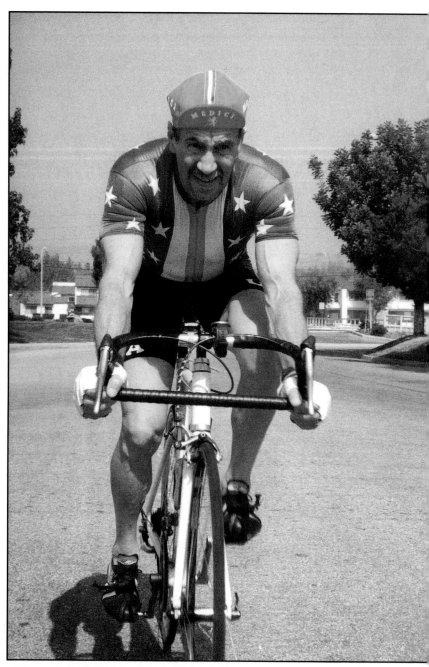

Phil Guarnaccia's innovative fitness program for his company has been studie
by experts both from the U.S. and abroad.

Joseph Hauser, Jr., has won more than 120 automobile races since 1969.

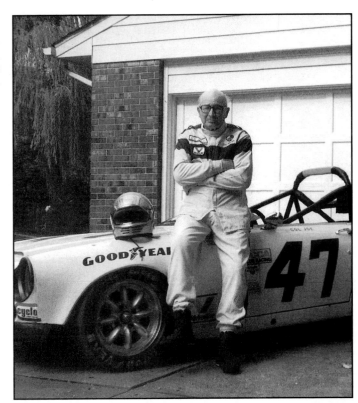

Henninges is one
el racer who loves
horses *almost* as
ch as she loves her
dren!

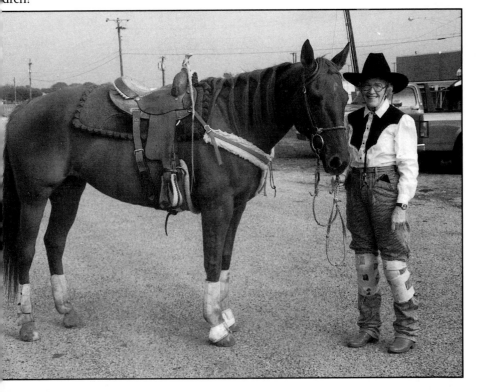

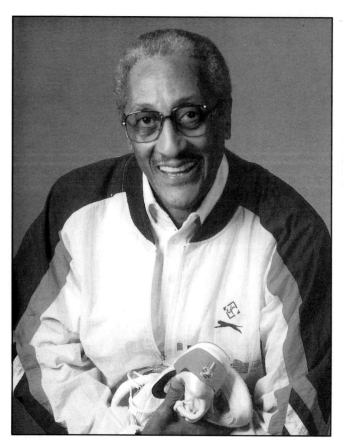

When Jim Law decided t| get in shape, he lost an amazing 125 pounds in six months.

Roy Houston "Tuffy" Overturf would rather rope calves than just about anything.

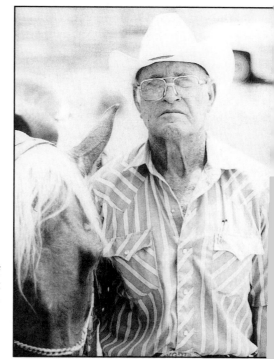

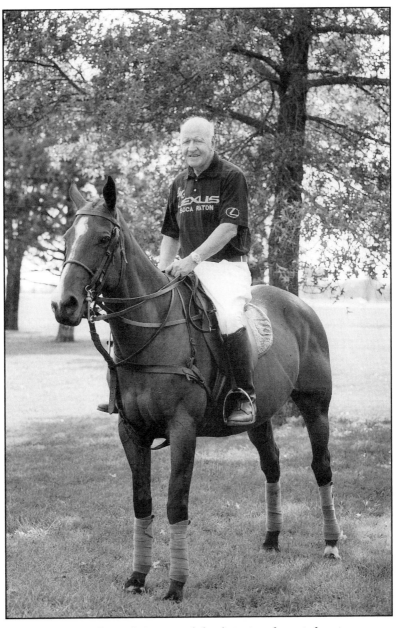

John T. Oxley still excels in one of the fastest and most dangerous sports in the world—polo.

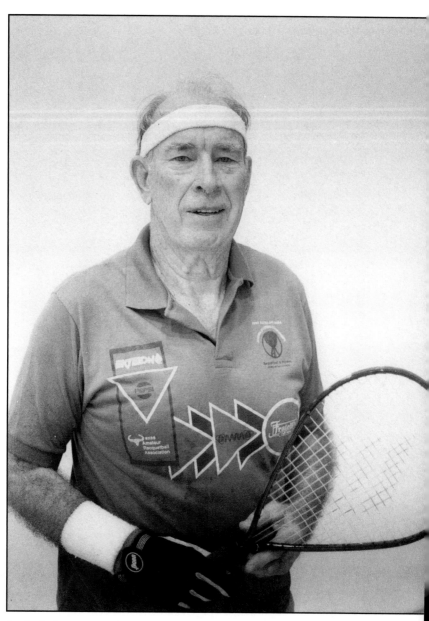

Joe Jack Pearce is as fanatical about fitness for seniors as he is about racquetba

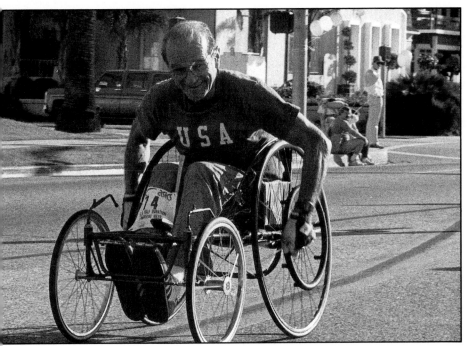

eelchair marathon specialist Max Rhodes is a national hero in Japan.

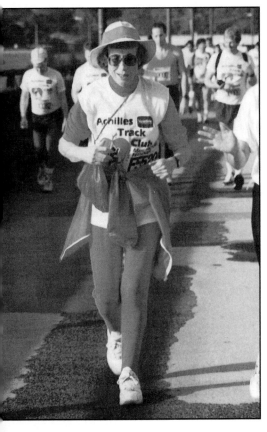

Lois Schieffelin runs the New York Marathon both because it makes her feel good and because of all of the great delis she discovers along the way.

Dr. Eugene L. Shirk is not only the oldest active college coach in America, he's one of the most successful.

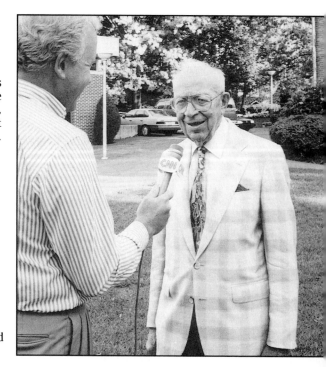

Esther Slager still has the style and grace that earned her the U.S.O. title of "Miss Foxhole of 1942."

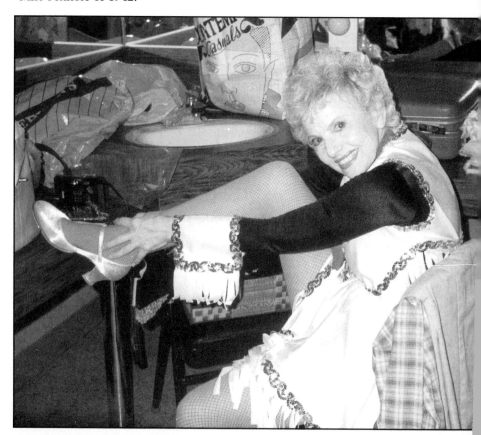

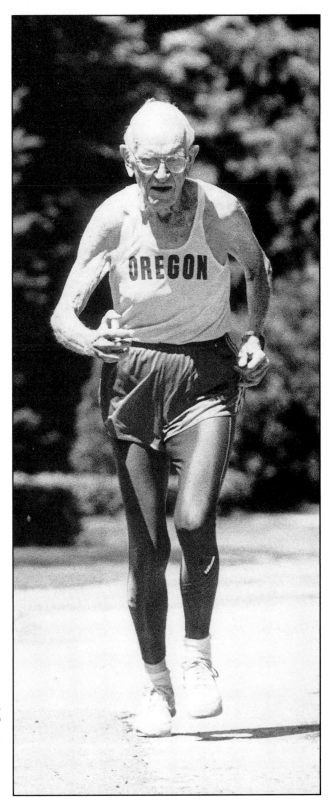

Dr. Paul Spangler has held more than 200 running records.

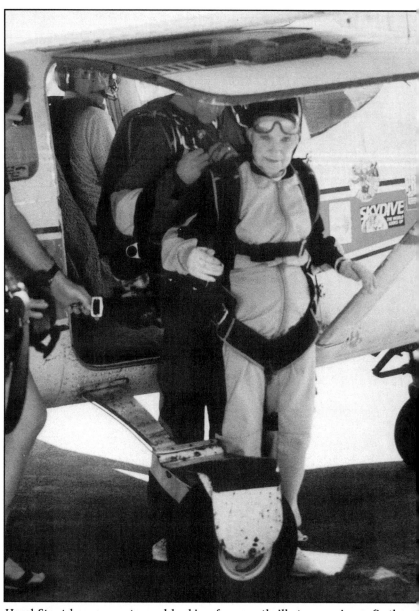

Hazel Stout has never stopped looking for new thrills to experience firsthand

Virginia "Ginnie" Wagner is a member of the famed "Dancin' Grannies" aerobic dance team.

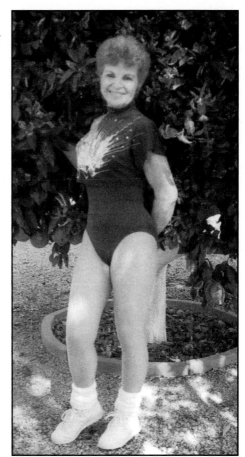

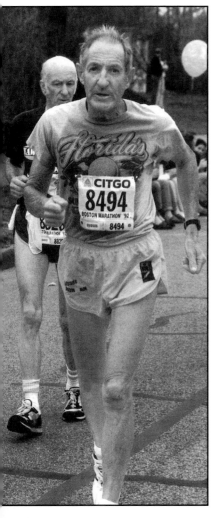

Jim Ward is a war hero who turned to the grueling Ironman Triathlon—for fun!

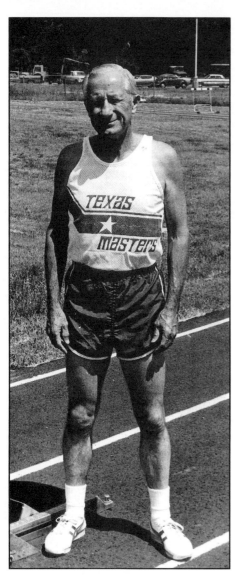

Dr. Fred White has won 250 gold medals
a sprinter and is aiming for that many m

Dexter Woodford is one of
America's best senior swimmers.

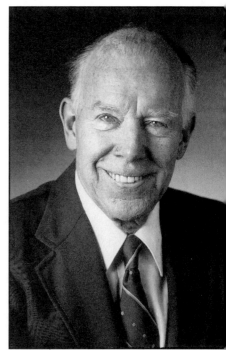

Chapter 14

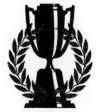

John T. Oxley

BOCA RATON, FLORIDA—At 83, John T. Oxley is the oldest polo player in the world still actively competing. The self-made millionaire has had a lifetime of thrills from playing what many consider to be the fastest—and most dangerous—team sport on the planet.

Playing polo successfully, Oxley believes, requires total commitment and total concentration.

"You're on a 1,100-pound horse going 30–35 mph, and you've got seven other players out there. You've got to use a lot of anticipation for the next play. The timing of the hand/eye contact, everything in fact, has to be perfect," he said. "That takes concentration. You've got balls three-and-a-quarter inches in diameter and you've got a three-quarter inch surface on the head of the mallet to hit it.

"I've played all the sports and polo is the toughest game of all. Nothing compares to this as far as fun and the challenge to try to be better. There's just something about it. It's just more difficult to do. I guess that's one of the attractions. It's just plain dangerous; polo requires a lot of risk. There have been a number of fatalities. You don't go out there to get killed—but, hey!—it's possible. That's where the concentration comes in."

How good is John's concentration? In 1970, he took his entire team to England to compete in the British Gold Cup world polo championships. In a practice game before the championship round, somebody knocked John and his horse over the boards, injuring John.

"That threw my back out on the second lumbar in the tailbone," he said. "The disk went over and began irritating the sciatic nerve. Well, in polo, you ride your horse from your thighs, from your knees up, really, so I was in pain.

"I went to the bone doctor in Tulsa. He said, 'You'd better take me along with you to see to that damage.' I said, 'I can't afford you!' So he gave me some pills and I took the pills—but they got to where they didn't help me through the tournament. I even went to a chiropractor and that didn't help."

At last, the pain was so great—and the match so close—that John sent his wife to buy boxes of Ace bandages.

"She wrapped my thigh from my crotch down to my knee as tight as she could, then put *another* one over it," he said. "It cut off about three-fourths of the circulation, but that killed a lot of the pain. And I got through the semi-finals and the finals on that basis. We won, becoming the first American team to win. I would say that was probably a highlight."

Now, *that's* concentration.

It is the single-minded concentration on achieving a goal that's marked John T. Oxley's life since his days as a boy on an Oklahoma cattle ranch.

"I was on a horse, I guess, every day from age three on up," he said. "I rode to school five-six miles every day, until I went away to college. I had to quit college after about five months when Dad called up and said, 'I've lost the ranch, all the cattle, and everything we have.' That happened when cattle went to five cents a pound and they foreclosed on him. So I had to go to work."

John went to work for an oil company, first as a bookkeeper, eventually—years later—as an owner. Through it all, he retained his love for horses.

"That's what attracted me to this polo game," he said. "My wife and I courted in the 4,000-acre park in Tulsa on horseback. Then we happened to run across a polo game they were playing there one Sunday. Will Rogers was playing in that game, incidentally. I talked to the captain of one of the teams and asked how I could learn the game because I wanted to play it someday. I think I was about 23 or 24 then.

"But I got real busy in business, raising a family, and building a couple of large corporations—and decided I didn't have time."

In the years ahead, John amassed a fortune in oil. But the cost was an inordinate amount of time spent in the air and the stress that comes from winning and losing millions on a single oil well.

Eventually, he returned to polo as an outlet.

"A friend of mine who had played polo all of his life in Santa Barbara called and said, 'John, when are you going to quit talking about playing polo and start playing?' I said, 'I think it is about time. What do you have in mind?' He said, 'We've got a top trainer out here, the best I've ever seen at training polo ponies. I think you ought to fly out here and hire him!'

"So we made an appointment, flew out to Santa Barbara, had dinner with him, and I hired him to get me mounted and started in polo. This was 1956, and I was 46 years old. I almost put it off too long, but I've had a lot of fun."

John tried to cram his rapidly increasing interest in polo into a schedule that included running a number of successful companies. It didn't work. Polo always finished second.

"I tried to retire at age 53 when I sold a large corporation back in 1962," he said. "I told my wife, 'I've worked hard all of my life, 14 hours a day, seven days a week, I think I'll just retire.' We started traveling around the country. We went to Santa Barbara and almost bought a home there. Then we went to Kentucky and I almost bought a thoroughbred breeding farm there—but that deal didn't come through for some reason.

"Finally, we came back to Tulsa, Oklahoma, my headquarters. By then my son had finished graduate school in geology. I said, 'Son, you're not dry behind the ears yet, but come on down and I'm going to teach you the oil business.' So we started yet another company in 1962. And pretty soon we had another large company again."

Finally, the polo bug got the best of him and became the dominant interest in his life (although he still runs two of his companies). He moved to Boca Raton on a full-time basis, established the Royal Palm Polo Club, and began assembling a crack polo team, one that eventually included nine-goaler Juan Badiola of Argentina (Ten goals is the highest ranking possible, and only six players in the world have it).

"I represent Boca Raton Royal Polo Club," John said. "Right now we're sponsored by J.M. Lexus, who sells the Lexus car. We currently have a good team. We won the $100,000 National Gold Cup in 1991 and we got in the finals in 1992, but lost. We've won the Sunshine League about half the time since 1960 and have been to the national tournament nearly every year.

"The highlight of my career was winning the British Gold Cup in 1970. I shipped 38 thoroughbred horses over there and we beat 12 international teams. It was quite an affair. We weren't expected to win it."

The Boca Raton team includes players ranging from their early 20s to their late 30s—and John. Even though it is his team, players and commentators say that John carries his weight on the polo field. He currently is a one-goaler, although he has been as high as a four-goaler in his career.

"It's like any other sport—the earlier you start, the better you are," he said. "The young guys can get it up to seven, eight, or nine goals, if they start real young. My two sons got up to five goals in their teens. Now they're businessmen. The average businessman can't make over a five- or six-goals handicap. The professionals play every day all the time, they're on horses all day long, and studying the game all week. It's like an amateur basketball player versus a professional. "Down in Argentina, they start some kids at seven–eight years of age, and they've turned out more high-goal polo players than we have here in the States. Most of our boys have to work part of the day and many of the Argentinians don't do anything but play."

Still, John's presence causes something of a commotion wherever he plays. Neither the Argentinians nor the British, the two most polo-crazy nations in the world, have ever had a tournament player over the age of 40.

"Everybody thinks I'm crazy, but I don't feel that way about it," John said. "It has been a catalyst to me and a challenge. I lost my beautiful wife four years ago and I think if I hadn't had this sport—and got myself busy in business—I probably would have committed suicide.

"It's a challenge, just like business has been. Getting out there, trying to win. To me, winning isn't the only thing, it's everything. If that's your goal, go for it. If it is starting out in business and having a goal of making a million dollars—I believe if you work hard enough at it, whatever it is, it'll come.

"It's like everything else—you plan the game before you ever go on the field. You need proper players, proper horses, proper teamwork and you'll go from there."

Not that success has come easily, of course. To maintain the level of physical fitness needed to compete on an international level, John has a vigorous daily workout routine.

"On a training day, I do aerobics for 20–25 minutes in the morning when I get up," he said. "Evenings before dinner I get on the bedroom rug and do it again. I try to ride as much as possible, although I don't make it every day. I play polo two or three times a week. And I try to walk two–three miles a day. So

I've got a pretty heavy routine, but that's what I attribute my longevity to as much as anything.

"Secondly, I've never had a heavy diet. I had a beautiful wife who knew how to fix lovely vegetables and fruit. We'd have steak or fish once a week and that's stayed about the same. I don't eat heavily. For lunch for years now I've had—while running two large corporations—a slice of whole-wheat bread with peanut butter on it, several slices of onions, and a glass of buttermilk. That's still my lunch every day. I just love onions.

"In the '60s, a friend of mine said, 'John, why don't you smoke a cigar after you make one of these big deals?' I said, 'OK.' I smoked for about four or five years, then I decided it was a dirty habit. So in 1970, after I'd finished winning the Gold Cup in England, I told my wife I'd never smoke any more cigars. I threw them all away and never smoked again. I've never smoked a cigarette in my life, never took a drink until 35. I've tried to live a clean life—as much as possible."

Of course, no amount of physical fitness can guarantee an injury-free career, especially in a sport as potentially dangerous as polo. Still, other than the back and nerve problem in 1970, John had never had a major injury in polo until 1990.

"A fellow was playing with long reins and the toe of my boot jerked the reins out of his hands. He jerked them back up into the air, and I fell six and a half feet," John said. "I broke seven ribs—the top one in two places—punctured my right lung, pinched a nerve in my shoulder, and later developed a nerve problem in my right hand.

"It took me three or four months to get over all of that."

Unfortunately, John's overall health picture hasn't been as pain-free. In the winter of 1983, he felt a tightness in his chest while playing polo. That spring he went to the Mayo Clinic and had an angiogram.

"The doctor called me at noon that day and said 'Mr. Oxley, we did 18 angiograms this morning and we've got four bad ones. Yours is one of them. We don't want you to leave the room this afternoon. We're going to do a bypass on you.'

"So I sat down and wrote my son a five-page letter, then told the doctor, 'Go to it.' That afternoon I had a triple bypass.

"I asked them later what caused it. And they said, 'Well, a lot of people talk about cholesterol. We think this one is 85 percent stress and 15 percent cholesterol. We think you've led a stressful life in business.'"

Which he had. John had started with nothing and had

built an oil-based empire that spanned the country. Along the way he'd owed banks tens of millions of dollars and had paid his debts. He would routinely do a couple of $10–15 million deals in a day.

"So I asked the doctors, 'How come I didn't have a heart attack?'" John recalled. "The doctors said, 'Well, your left ventricle was 85 percent plugged up and your right ventricle is twice as large as it should be, so it is carrying twice the blood it should carry. It was just carrying it over to the left side of your heart, which is why you never had a heart attack. That's due to your physical activity all of your life.'"

Since that time, John has gone to the Mayo Clinic twice a year for a complete physical.

"I take a treadmill every year and, at my age, I asked them how many minutes I was supposed to take on it. They said, 'Three-and-a-half minutes or more at your age.' And they ran me up to 13 minutes!

"Then they put you on a bike, put a camera on your chest, put dye in your bloodstream, tie all of that to a computer, and measure the flow of blood through all of your arteries. Three years ago, the two guys running it said I checked out like someone about 55 years of age. The next year, the guy said I checked out at about 50 years of age! I said, 'If I keep coming back, will I get down to 21?'"

Through it all, John says his doctors have been supportive of his high degree of physical activity.

"About a year or two ago, my doctor said, 'John, I want you to keep up what you're doing. I've got a lot of patients who are 60–65 who are not as mentally alert as you are. Keep doing your business like you're doing. Secondly, keep up exercise and aerobics. Thirdly, I'd like to tell you to quit playing polo, but I know you're not going to do it. I will tell you that, if you have a fall, you're not going to heal as fast. Fourth, I want you to keep up your sex life.'

"I said, 'What has *that* got to do with anything?' He said, 'Well, it ties in with your hormones, testosterone, and those things that are just part of the body, and I want you to keep it up.'"

Today John says it is no secret how he continues to amaze onlookers and confound opposing polo players at age 83. You *must*—and he is adamant about the "must" part—keep active physically.

"I see people aged 55–65 at Mayo, walking through those halls, who've got not just one foot in the grave, they've got *both* feet in the grave," he said. "They're stooped over and they're physically shot, and I think it is all because they've led sedentary lives.

"I grew up in the oil business in Tulsa, which used to be the oil center of the world. All of the major oil companies are there and I have friends at all of them. They all had mandatory retirement at age 65. After retirement, they'd all start going over to the Petroleum Club where they'd start have lunch, play poker, and drink. Then they'd go home and have another drink. They were all gone in about five years, too. I don't have any pallbearers left. I think if they had kept active, they'd still be alive.

"But as for me, I'm going to keep playing polo. I'm going to let them carry me out with my boots on."

Do these sound like the words of an optimistic, positive person?

"Oh, I think so," John agreed firmly. "I always took the attitude that you could do most anything you made up your mind to do. It just takes a little longer sometimes. I believe in stick-to-itiveness and persistence when you meet resistance. If I had to define success, I'd say 'Work, work, work. Persistence, persistence, persistence. And good common sense.'"

Isn't that something of a contradiction in terms? Polo and common sense? What is so compelling about the sport that forces an 83-year-old to risk life and limb—and fortune—to play polo with men 50 years his junior?

To a polo purist, of course, the answer is obvious.

"Polo is like baseball," he said. "You play sandlot baseball and when you move up to majors, there's no comparison. Polo's the same way. You can play low ball polo and play with your older guys, your slower guys, but it is just not the game I call polo.

"*Real* polo is so challenging. You've got to do the right thing and do it quickly. You've got to control your horse, you've got to anticipate the next play, you've got to ride off the younger guys—just bump the hell out of them!—and it is an entirely different game than with older players. It is hockey on horseback."

Having said all of that, it is not surprising that John suggests that polo is the perfect sport, *especially* for the young person who wants to be playing polo as well as John—or wants to at least be as active and vital as John—when he or she reaches the age of 83.

"I would tell him to set up a physical routine and stick with it every day, exercise every day, and ride as much as he possibly could," John said. "First, to become a good polo player, you've got to become a good horseman. I would tell him to ride, ride, ride everyday until he got so tired that he relaxed from the waist down. You've got to develop light hands since a polo pony has a light mouth and because we ask them to do a lot of things. You can't play if you've got heavy hands on the bridle. And develop a good seat and keep working at it just like anything else. Spend as much time as you possibly can with it."

But what if you're no longer 25? What if you're 45 or 55 or even 65? What if you're looking at retirement age and you see John T. Oxley on the polo pony, apparently as lean and as supple as the young men around him?

"What can I do?" you ask. "Is it too late for me to play polo?"

"I would certainly encourage you to go ahead, although I would tell you it is more difficult to get up to my status and handicap at your age," he said carefully. "I think I encourage a lot of guys to start at ages 45–50. And they have, and they've had a lot of fun. Of course, it helps if they've already learned to ride before they start."

John is living proof of his words. He's become a living legend in polo circles, a white-haired, ruddy-cheeked, grim-eyed avenger, a great-grandfather with an eye for the goal.

How do we know? Because Boca Raton's star player, 31-year-old Juan Badiola, says so.

"I go back to Buenos Aires and show films of our matches to friends," Badiola told *The New York Times*. "I say, 'See that fellow there, he is 83 years old.' They can't believe it. They say, 'Eighty-three years old, and he still gets on a horse? Incredible!'"

Or ask some of the top polo players in England. In 1990, John returned to the English Gold Cup, although strictly as an observer this time.

"Some of the lords we'd played against in 1970 came up and said, 'My God, John, you're still alive *and* still playing polo! We can't believe it!'"

Finally, *The New York Times* once estimated it cost John half a million dollars a year to field his team.

"Polo is addictive," he told *The Times*, "and the only two ways I know to get out of it are to go broke or die. And I'm not either, yet."

Chapter 15

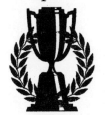

Joe Jack Pearce

WACO, TEXAS—At the Waco Family YMCA, Joe Jack Pearce is all business. It's lunch time and Joe Jack and his 55-year-old partner are in a fast and furious racquetball game with a couple of opponents half their age. A handful of people gather around the challenge court to watch the action.

Finally, one of the younger players sends a backhand shot rocketing past both Joe Jack and his friend. The two older men have lost, but just barely. The other two stand with their hands on their knees.

Joe Jack pounds one on the back. "Hey! How about a rematch?"

The younger men demur. One mumbles something about getting back to work and he heads for the showers. Joe Jack shrugs his muscular shoulders and begins a rhythmic pounding of the racquetball against the far wall.

At age 82, Joe Jack Pearce is the world champion racquetball player in his age bracket. He's also nationally ranked in a number of track and field events.

For Joe Jack, fitness and health are lifelong obsessions.

"I think we Americans as a people are grossly ignorant on the structure and function of our bodies," he said. "We will, for instance, accept a nostrum advertised on TV as a cure for what we think we have, whether it is arthritis or ptomaine poisoning or whatever. We will self-medicate without actually knowing what's happening, what can happen with the human body.

"Instead, we need to know that it is exercise that is necessary. The body is made to work."

Joe Jack was one of five boys, the sons of a Southern Baptist preacher.

"Three of us boys were active in athletics from high school on," he said. "Growing up, we moved between small Texas towns, from Westminster to Sherman to Farmersville. It was in Farmersville that I went to high school. It was a small school and four of us finished there. All five of us grew up to be schoolteachers."

Joe Jack's high school football teams at Farmersville won both bi-district and regional championships in 1927 and 1928. Like his brothers, Joe Jack also competed in basketball and track. Three of the brothers also eventually ran track at Baylor University.

"I went to Baylor in December 1930, after attending Burleson Junior College, which closed in December 1930," he said. "I finally found a job, a place to eat, and a place to sleep. I became eligible for athletics at Baylor in the fall of 1931, but my job played out and I had to drop out of school. I went back in the fall of 1932 and played football and ran track."

Actually, Joe Jack's football career was a little more exciting than that. Halfway through the 1933 season, the Baylor coach shifted him to quarterback. The team promptly won its next five games and Joe Jack was named to several All-American teams.

After graduation, he took a coaching job in the small town of Edna in south Texas, between Houston and San Antonio.

"We had a little town softball team back then and I was on the town basketball team," he recalled. "When you're coaching, you normally don't like to see yourself going to pot, so I stayed in fair shape—just maintaining my physical condition as best I could to coach and to demonstrate and to do things."

World War II interrupted Joe Jack's coaching career. Three of the Pearce boys joined the Army Air Corps, while Joe Jack went into the Navy.

After the war, he coached four more years in Beeville. Eventually he came to the Waco Independent School District as director of health and physical education, but without any coaching responsibilities.

It was in Waco that Joe Jack discovered racquetball. It was love at first carom. From that point on, he played tirelessly whenever he had a spare moment.

"In 1970, I heard of Senior Olympics, Inc.," he said. "There were 42 sports in it back then. In 1972, when I was 62, I went out to Los Angeles to participate.

"The next year racquetball was introduced to the games, so I took a weekend of my vacation time and went out and played racquetball. I'd stay the week, then participate in the track and field events the second weekend. I did that for about three years.

"And then came the Texas Senior Olympics, later called the Texas Senior Games. I've been participating in the Texas Senior Games in racquetball and track and field ever since—although more field than track."

Joe Jack retired from the Waco school district at age 66 and began helping underprivileged children at his church's activities center. The rest of the time he devoted to the racquetball tournament circuit.

He was an immediate success. Today, his closets are crammed full of the trophies and medals he's won both in racquetball and track and field. He is currently the world champion in racquetball in the 80-plus age bracket. He is also ranked first in Texas in the 75-plus, and second in the country in the 75-plus bracket for the same sport.

"I don't know if I was just tenacious or what, but when I first started playing racquetball, they didn't have a bracket older than 45-plus, so I played the kids!" he said. "It was years before I got into even a 65-plus age bracket. Now we've grown to 75-plus and there will be other brackets added in the years ahead."

Joe Jack's first national title was in the 75-plus bracket in Houston in the late 1980s, and that championship still has a special place on his wall. But his favorite memory is from an early Senior Olympics week in Los Angeles.

"Going to another part of the country, like Los Angeles where they're sports-minded, and competing with people who have grown up in track and field and racquetball and coming from a state that's really a foreign country to them and tanning their hides in racquetball and doing fairly well with the other activities is another achievement that I am proud of.

"Also, at Syracuse at the National Senior Sports Classic in the summer of 1992, I entered a number of events. The ages ranged from 55-up to 100-plus. We had one or two who were in the 100-year-old bracket. I competed in five events in the 80–84 age bracket and I placed in all five of them. I got a fourth place in the horseshoes, second place in the javelin, third place in the shot put, fifth in the discus, and sixth in the high jump.

"There was a new world record in the 80-plus set in the high jump. A man jumped four feet, one inch. So all of that was special as well."

Joe Jack will be returning to Baton Rouge in June 1993 and

will participate in the same events (save for the high jump), along with racquetball, which will become an official sport there for the first time in '93.

Incidentally, Joe Jack has another unusual "first" in his life. In July 1972, Jackie Sorenson came to the University of Texas in Austin to teach instructors of aerobic dance. Joe Jack believes he was the first certified male instructor *ever* in aerobic dance.

Still, despite his successes elsewhere, racquetball remains his first love. But he says it has as much to do with the competition and camaraderie as it does with the physical aspects of the sport.

"I guess in tournament play I learned early on that when I got into the Seniors, the 50-plus, that I was in with a group of men who were highly professional people," he said. "They were top individuals, this was the highest class of athletes that I had ever associated with. And I still feel this way about this senior group."

Maintaining his level of fitness is a full-time job, Joe Jack says. He avoids spicy foods, but eats a regular, well-balanced diet.

"I haven't changed my diet at all," he said, "although sometimes I'm over-nutritioned and over-fed. At those times I'll go to much smaller meals. And I have gone to a diet four–five times over the years to reduce the girth. Otherwise, I have just a regular diet. I believe you shouldn't let your girth get too far out because this puts an extra load on your heart, and it puts a great load on your knees and hip joints.

"I also smoked coming through high school and during World War II. Come training time for athletics, though, we cut it out. We had a coach in high school who was rigid in his training rules and we respected him a great deal. He said, 'Do this and you'll be successful.'"

Joe Jack said he still abides by many of the rules first outlined by his high school coach.

"He said, 'You've got to take care of yourself physically before the game, during the game, and after the game because you've got to play next week. You've got to take care of yourself.' So I still don't abuse any habit of work or play, whatever the sport."

But he also admits that his robust physique may be due, in part, to genetics.

"I had uncles who lived to be in their late 90s. They were in good shape up past 90," he said. "My mother, at the time of her death at 86, was active and agile. She was in church work, in politics, and she was just as alert as she had always been. My father died of a heart attack when he was 70."

To stay in shape, Joe Jack has a regular workout routine, including a time of what he calls "strength maintenance."

"In my training, I never take more than a 35-pound weight in each hand, and I do most of it with 20 or 25 pounds," he said. "I do exercises that work towards the development of a specific need or skill. I have an objective. I may want to increase my distance on the shot put or javelin or discus.

"I do weight training to maintain or to increase some areas. Sometimes when I'm playing, I find out that my shoulders or my thighs are a little weaker than I want, so when I get back and start training, I'll build those parts of the body up with exercise. The way I train is to work on the deficiencies. It's a continual process. I work out five days a week; I do weights three or four times a week."

Joe Jack's sole physical ailment—save for a broken collarbone in high school—came following his six-week trip to compete in the Senior Games in Syracuse, New York.

"We had a new van. When I got back from driving that van and holding on to that steering wheel, I had tendinitis so bad I had two hooks for hands and pain in my shoulder, too," he said. "I went to orthopedic people and they told me what it was and that I'd probably have it from now on at my age. It was months before I could grasp a weight to do any upper-arm and body-strength training. I couldn't hold my racquetball racquet, so from July to January I didn't do anything but walk and run and lower extremity exercises. It has been difficult to get back in shape. But I knew ahead of time if I didn't exercise—at my age—I'd never get back to any standard."

Despite the bout with tendinitis, Joe Jack says his family doctors have been supportive of his intense level of physical activity.

"Now, there was one doctor—I was playing basketball with a team in Beeville after the war when I was about 40—who told me, 'You'll have to quit playing basketball as hard as you play it because you're getting old enough now that you need to go to something else.' But I stayed active anyway. And I haven't had a thorough physical examination by a physician, other than for shots and blood pressure checks, since 1963! I don't traipse in and out of a doctor's office very often."

Joe Jack believes that there is a close connection between the spiritual and physical sides of a person.

"In a game, in any activity, there are rules," he said. "To me, the written rule in a game is to be followed to a 'T.' As far as I'm concerned, I expect to play according to the rules as written. And then, if someone shows me that my interpretation of the rules is incorrect, I'll make some kind of a change.

"I think that ought to be true of us in living, too. God gave us this body; He gives us lots of things that we don't look after. But if we don't look after this body, then we don't have much left to show people!"

Beyond racquetball, Joe Jack and his wife Mary Catherine's favorite pastimes include travelling across the United States and Canada and attending their grandchildrens' baseball, basketball, and soccer games whenever possible.

But he admits that watching someone else participate in a sporting event can be frustrating.

"I didn't realize that I was as much of a stickler for form and skill as I am," he said. "But as I watch these kids at the Little League fields playing ball, and I watch them at the basketball games, their coaches are not paying attention to the physical skill and technique of the participants. They're not watching the stance of the batter, they don't watch the way he handles the ball and whether he can throw with his right hand or left hand.

"People need to pay more attention to skill development and strength maintenance to execute a particular skill at a high level. This doesn't come through a one-day-a-week workout or by only thinking about it. It takes some attention. It takes some work. It takes some concentration."

Joe Jack's high visibility has also meant that people approaching retirement age often seek him out for advice on how to remain active past the age of 65—or even how to do as well as he does when they reach 82.

"To get to this level, it would depend on their physique," he said. "I meet many people like this, (and my admonition to them is this: 'Find something you want to do *before* you retire and begin to learn about it. Don't leave this gap in here. Get a target, a goal, to work on.

"I would encourage seniors to be involved in some kind of exercise which has a resistance to it, whether weight lifting, or just lifting a chair, pressing against the floor, even doing sit-ups."

He is quick to suggest a gradual increase in activity, however, particularly for those seniors who begin a program to restore physical fitness late in life.

"You have to be careful," Joe Jack said. "If you go into it too strong—and I've seen people do this—you'll strain a muscle, injure a joint. Some run too soon and too long on hard surfaces. I tell them to walk before they run, to guard against injuries. Do not expect to get into shape the first week, the first month, the first year, even. Do it gradually and be satisfied with each point in your development, but do not, do *not* over-stress your heart, your muscles, or your joints. Because this is a time when osteoporosis is in the picture. You can injure a joint that may not be replaceable or correctable. So be careful."

Still, he stresses that sore or stiff muscles are *not* an acceptable reason to refrain from exercise altogether. It is, he says, simply too important.

"If you're sore, instead of running on the pavement or running around the track, do what we call in physical education 'passive manipulation.' Lie down on your back and work your legs like you are running. Or do your push-ups one hand against the other to gain strength.

"That's how people give up exercise. They say, 'I hurt, I can't do it today. I'll do it tomorrow.' Well, tomorrow comes and they still can't do it. And on the third day, they say, 'Well, I feel so good, I don't think I'll do *any* work or exercise today.' And finally, it just goes away from them."

Joe Jack's particular concern, however, is for seniors who have spent most of their lives in a sedentary manner.

"Exercise is not always comfortable or convenient," he said. "If seniors would just think. 'What else am I going to do with my time that would be better for me than exercise?' There are clubs, YMCAs, church facilities—all have programs for seniors and someone to supervise these programs. I would encourage them to get with other people in these kinds of exercises. And I would highly recommend resistance exercises, like weight training.

"It is *never* too late if one will enter into it with a spirit of 'I want to achieve.'"

Still, Joe Jack said he never imagined when he began actively competing in racquetball at age 67 that he would someday become the 80-plus world champion.

"In fact, there wasn't an 80-plus category when I started in racquetball!" he said with a laugh. "I'm the champion in 80-plus because I've been in it this long and have learned to play it this well.

"When somebody first comes out of the 70-plus bracket, they might beat the tar out of me because I'm 82—there's a five-year age bracket here. I'm not about to think I can come down to the 'Y' and beat a good 25-year-old or even a 45-year-old racquetball player when he's in good shape and I'm in good shape, because his skills are different. He's quicker, his reactions, his anticipation are different.

"But just realize where you are, and be satisfied and happy with yourself."

At the same time, there are a host of 35-year-old racquetball players at the YMCA in Waco who would be satisfied and happy if Joe Jack Pearce would stick to playing and beating men his *own* age!

Chapter 16

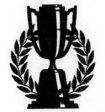

Maxime Rhodes

MIAMI, FORIDA—In 1969, Maxime Arrista Rhodes was sitting pretty. The 56-year-old Navy veteran was making a good living selling real estate in Miami. He had four kids, a nice house, a comfortable life. He pretty much had it all.

One typically splendid Florida morning, he took his ladder to the front yard to trim some palm tree fronds that were hanging over the sidewalk.

"I was on the top of a high ladder when the bottom slipped out," Max said. "I broke my back and severed my spinal cord."

Max never walked again.

Flash forward to 1991. It is the 11th National Veterans Wheelchair Games. Max has just received the prestigious "Spirit of the Games" award, given to the athlete who "most epitomizes the qualities of a champion—athletic excellence, sportsmanship and character."

As recipient of the award, Max received a free trip to Washington D.C., met then–Vice President Dan Quayle, toured the White House, and sat in the review stand for the Fourth of July parade.

Today, 80-year-old Max is the unchallenged champion of the senior wheelchair marathon. The 1993 Boston Marathon will be his 80th marathon. He is the current world record holder with one epic 62-mile pull in a wheelchair.

Max was born in rural Virginia in 1913. There were only 15 in his tiny high school class. He was selected as all-county forward in basketball his senior year, but rarely played again.

"I was born in the deep Depression," he said. "I left the farm and went to drive a truck, then joined the National Guard to get an extra one dollar a week for two years. Later I decided to go to Chicago because my mother was originally from up that way. So I thought it would be good to go there someday.

"When I went to Chicago, it was the World's Fair time, but I was not able to get a job there. I hung on anyway, and finally got jobs as a theater usher at night and a golf course caddy during the day. After about a year, I was able to get into the country club to wash windows and things like that."

Eventually, Max saved enough money to buy a few trucks and get married. Just when his fledgling trucking business was booming, World War II broke out. When the time came, Max chose the Navy and immediately shipped out.

"In the Navy, I was a mechanic," he said. "We originally had two refrigeration men, but we lost them and no one knew anything about coding systems. So when the equipment came in, I said, 'I'd rather try this than go out with the boats.' I was able to follow the instructions and so, when the walk-in coolers and ice machines came in, I was a popular guy! I did real well and I moved up to First Class."

Max saw action in the South Pacific near Saipan and Tinian. He was still on Tinian when the end came with a couple of violent, mushroom-shaped clouds.

"I was on Tinian from the time we took it over," he said. "I was there when they launched the atomic bomb, although we didn't know it until we heard about it over the radio at 8 a.m. When the *Enola Gay*, the plane that took the first bomb to Hiroshima returned, the whole island turned out to see it. There were so many people there at the air base who wanted to see it, they held us back until the crew got out. Then we were allowed to go touch it and take pictures of it.

"That happened in August 1945. There were so many soldiers and sailors to get back to the United States, I didn't get back until December."

Alas, like many vets, Max wasn't sure what to do when he returned.

"Before I left I was in the trucking business and I was up to seven trucks," he said. "But I had to give that up to go in the service. So my wife—at that time—had to take over. That was disastrous—she didn't know much about trucks."

Max lost it all. He then went to work selling appliances. He did so well that in two years he opened an appliance store of his own!

"I became a retailer selling refrigerators in Arlington Heights, Illinois," Max said. "I hung around Chicago for about 20 years.

I had three stores, then I consolidated them in a big building I had built out in the country. We were able to triple the business in the new store and it went real well. I sold it out in '58 and had enough money to move to Florida."

Max chose the Miami area and used the money from the sale of his store to move into real estate and real estate management. Once again, he did well.

Then came the accident and the years of rehabilitation. But the same man who had washed windows and driven cabs for a living in Depression-era Chicago was not about to allow a small thing like a wheelchair to slow him down.

"At that time I had two apartment buildings and six stores," he said. "I sold them all to a fellow I had met, but he wanted me to manage them, and I've done that ever since. I've got my little office here and I oversee eight units in one building, six in another, and six stores—they're all together in one big complex."

In 1974, Max began to take advantage of the services offered at a nearby veterans hospital. It was then that he first heard about the National Veterans Wheelchair Games. He was amazed when, a few years later, a couple of acquaintances returned from the Richmond, Virginia, games with chests full of medals.

"I couldn't believe it!" Max said. "They were telling me, 'You could be in there.' I said, 'I'm too old. I'm 68.' But I was exercising and they encouraged me to go.

"The next one was the following year in Milwaukee. So I just drove up there myself to see what it was all about because I hadn't seen what activities they had. What intrigued me was the basketball and the short races on the track.

"In 1982, I finally decided to enter the games in California and I signed up for swimming and a few other events—but not racing. When they talked to me at that time, I said 'I would like to try track.'

"Finally, in 1984 they talked me into racing and I got into it, but mostly short races on the track. Then they began telling me about the marathons and 10Ks and I said, 'I'll never be able to do that.'"

But the idea of competing in a marathon continued to haunt him. Just in case he *might* ever decide to try one, Max gradually upped his daily distance.

"In January 1985, they had a marathon in Miami and I really practiced for that; I was ready to go," he said. "I did real well and that really got me going. I had a lot of attention because of my age. Here I was, this 72-year-old guy in the midst of all these kids. So from there on I've liked the long distances."

Max says that his first marathon in Miami remains one of the most memorable.

"There was a wheelchair racer named Jim Knaub there, the greatest 'pusher,' as we call wheelchair racers, of his time," Max said. "I was 72. He won the race but heard about me and talked to me. He said, 'I can't believe it—I just can't believe it. Would you come to Long Beach, California, if we pay your expenses?' I said, 'Yeah, sure I would.' So in February they paid my air fare and hotel and that was my second marathon. That was a good race.

"I did a different marathon in Los Angeles a few months later, and while I was there, I talked to a gentleman who did the Boston Marathon. Everybody who does marathons talks Boston. The guy I talked to is in charge of the race in Boston. I got to him and introduced myself and I said, 'I would like to do the marathon in Boston.' He said, 'Well, maybe we can get you in.'

"I entered in 1986 and I've done Boston ever since. I recently wrote him and told him that I'd be 80 years old soon and I'd like to do my 80th marathon at Boston."

But it was a chance meeting in Los Angeles that eventually led to the biggest races—and most interesting experiences—of Max's life. During a post-race conversation with a young wheelchair racer, Max was told about the wheelchair-only marathon run annually in Oita, Japan. Intrigued by the prospect, Max entered the marathon, was accepted, flew to Japan, and participated in the race. It was love at first sight. In more ways than one.

"The first time I was there, I met Fumiko, the lady who served as interpreter. Fumiko has now been my wife for five years," Max said proudly.

The Japanese were enthralled with the gutsy American and have invited him back to Oita every year since 1985.

"The Governor of the city of Oita treats me like a son!" Max said. "He teases me and I tease him! The sponsors have paid my way to Japan, even in 1991 when I wasn't able to compete."

For the past three years, Max has been taking American T-shirts to students at Beppu Seishien (Handicapped Children's School) after the opening ceremonies. He had first noticed them lining the streets near Oita, encouraging the contestants in the marathon. Afterwards, he asked to meet them. Because of his work with the children, the marathon organizers recently presented Max with the Award of Merit of International Friendship.

"There's a boy in Japan who I race with over there every year. He began sending me T-shirts," Max said. "They are beautiful T-shirts that he makes himself. I wear them in the race in Japan.

"The day before the race they have a meeting in the big auditorium. It is translated into English and other languages because the wheelchair racers come from all over the world. Last year, there were 400 athletes from 38 countries represented in Oita. And there are no runners, just wheelchairs. It's a good thing.

"This will be their 12th marathon in 1992. It will be my seventh. I don't think any other foreigner has been that often. If they have, I haven't see them. They're not all there every year. The hotel, meals, and air fare are very expensive."

The only marathon Max missed was in 1991 when he had an accident before a race in Seattle and broke his hip.

"Of course I couldn't race, but I sent my application to Japan anyway and they said, 'Yes, you're coming,'" Max said. "They've always paid my expenses except for the first race."

And, oh yes, Fumiko does return to Japan with Max each year. She stays with her family for the weeks surrounding the race.

Actually, in the Miami area, Max is known for more than just his marathon accomplishments. For years, he has given unselfishly of his time and money to help young people in wheelchairs.

"I raised money for a girl I saw in a race about five years ago. She had a terrible chair," he said. "I started talking to her and asked her why and she said, 'Well, my parents are poor.' I liked the little girl, so I raised money and bought her a brand new chair.

"The mayor of Coral Cables heard my story. We had a little meeting, and after that I started a program for the kids. Since then we've taken in 77 wheelchair kids. I have old chairs donated to me and I have them re-done. I have five chairs of my own that I've done that with.

"These 77 kids came to a park near here with a track and I trained them as best I could. That's how it started off. I've got a little history on every one of them. A lot of those I trained now beat me in the races and marathons—and I love it! And some are going real good."

One of Max's protegées, Lisa Sandelin, also of Miami, recently became the first junior wheelchair competitor to finish a 50-mile race.

Max, incidentally, won that same 50-mile race with a time of six hours and seven minutes, despite the fact that he stopped for more than two minutes after 24 laps of the 26-lap event when he was mistakenly advised that he had completed the race!

Fifty miles in a wheelchair is not something that comes easily or naturally for anyone. Max says he has accomplished it with a regular exercise routine, a healthy diet, and supportive family, friends, and physicians.

"This morning I pushed six miles, blew a tire, and came in early," Max said. "The day before I did 10 miles. I try to go out every morning around 4–5 a.m. and I'm in by 6:30 a.m. That's how I do my practicing.

"I also have here in my little office a weight lift and a chin-up bar that I use every day."

His diet is supervised by wife Fumiko.

"She's wonderful," Max said. "She tells me exactly what I'm going to eat. She's very conscious of food. She's just wonderful; a chef couldn't do any better. And I pay attention to what she says.

"Before beginning in racing, I never ate a lot of meat. But since I've been married to Fumiko, she gives me a little meat with almost every meal. Not much, but I don't care much for meat. I'm very, very high on pie with ice cream, though!

"At one time I weighed 195 pounds, and now I'm only 142. When I started racing I was at 162. I got down to 130 and at that low weight I felt as though I might be weak, so I've added more food."

As for the moral support, Max says he's been fortunate in every aspect of his life.

"My doctors have always been pretty supportive," he said. "I'm only two miles from the VA Hospital and I just pop in there any time I've got a headache or anything. I'm always in pretty good health. Other than breaking my hip that time, I haven't been in the hospital. So my health is pretty good.

"There are a few of us around who are lucky to continue, who are in good health, who keep practicing, who take care of ourselves. For instance, I never smoked a cigarette after I was 20 years old. Now, my dad was smoking all the time and he was sick. The doctor told him, 'If you don't quit smoking, get yourself another doctor. Otherwise, you're going to die!'

"I took that as a sign that I needed to quit smoking. And I

never smoked again. My parents didn't really know I was smoking, anyway! And I'm sure that has helped me with my health—that I had brains enough to never smoke again."

Because of the physical benefits he's receiving from such a workout and competition schedule, Max says that he shares his fitness philosophy with anybody who will listen. His thesis? "It's never too late to get in shape."

"I tell young people, if they're able-bodied, to get in these short races," he said. "Start out, if you need to, in the walking section. It has gotten very popular here in Miami. That's what I tell them: exercise.

"Now for the people in their sixties who want to get in shape, I tell them to do just what I'm doing. The guys in the hospital, I *know* they're in bad shape, but if I could just get them into racing... You don't have to win—just participate. Somebody has to be last, but it doesn't matter. I explain that exercise is very, very important."

With that attitude, Max says winning has never been the reason he competes. Winning is just a small part of the whole package.

"That's why it doesn't bother me competing against the young guys," he said. "They're all kidding me, calling me 'dad' and 'ol' man.' They like to tease me and I like to be with them. But in the races and in the marathons, they just turn you loose. You can be as young as 14, and I'm always the oldest one.

"In the Veterans Games, there's a 40-and-above class where you become a master. So in those Games, I compete against the masters. Now, some of them say they don't want to be a master, especially guys in their 40s, 50s, even in their 60s. So far, though, there's nobody in their 70s! I've been to Europe, Canada, Japan. I've done marathons in Germany and Poland. I did a race in Poland that was 100K (62 miles) in 1987. It took me 10 hours. It was one of my highlights."

So, what's ahead for Max Rhodes? He says he doesn't plan very far in advance.

"Beyond my 80th marathon in Boston in '93, I'll just see how my health is," he said. "I don't know how much longer I'll marathon. It depends on my health."

If that's the case, then there is a little school for handicapped children in Japan, and a whole lot of people in the United States who each day wish Max a long life and good health.

Chapter 17

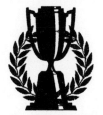

Lois Schieffelin

NEW YORK CITY—Each day, Lois Schieffelin jogs slowly, deliberately, through the streets of New York. At 81 years of age, she keeps an eye open for every possible hazard, from uncovered manholes in the Upper East Side, to racks of free-swinging clothes in the apparel district, to one of Gotham's legions of "characters" lurching towards her down a crowded sidewalk.

She also keeps an eye peeled for new delis, bargains, and out-of-the-way costume and theatrical supply shops. Lois is, after all, a true New Yorker.

Nothing deters Lois from her morning run. Not rain. Not the tourists and heat in August. Not even a recent hysterectomy.

As a result, she ran a personal best in the 1991 New York Marathon: 6 hours, 32 minutes, and 6 seconds. Lois also won the 1991 Abel Kiviat Award, named for a runner who had hoped to live to be 100, but died three months before his 100th birthday. The award is given to the oldest man and oldest woman who finish the race.

Not that any of this will surprise anyone who knows Lois and her family. She comes from a long line of long-lived, vital people.

"Oh my, yes, I come from an active family," she said. "My father was an artist and used to go to Egypt every year to paint in the tombs. He went the year before he died—and he died at 89. My mother, who was several years younger, also died at 89. I'm the baby of the family. I have one sister who is 88 and another who is 90. We're all still going strong. My 88-year-old sister still travels all over the world."

Lois is widowed. Her husband, John J. Schieffelin, died in 1987, also at the age of 89. Schieffelin was in the Navy during

World War I and became a Naval Aviator. He taught flying during World War II and eventually retired as a Rear Admiral.

The Schieffelins had one son, John J. Schieffelin, Jr., now 55. One of Lois' grandsons, John Clifford ("Jake") Schieffelin, followed in his grandfather's footsteps both by running marathons and by joining the Navy.

In fact, it was Lois and grandson Jake who convinced John Jr. to continue the family tradition.

"We had a terrible time persuading my son to run in the New York Marathon with us, but finally we bullied him into it," Lois said, without a hint of remorse. "John has now run 14 marathons, including Boston, and now loves it. It was Jake who kept urging me to run a marathon. He said he wanted three generations to run in the New York Marathon and he eventually got his way."

Still, marathon running was a fairly recent development in Lois' busy life. For many years, her great love was tennis.

"But as I got older, I found that the people who were beating me were the same ones I used to beat," she said. "And that really depressed me. Still, I always had a lot of fun.

"I once even qualified to play at the tournament at Forest Hills. Of course, that meant I drew Helen Jacobs, who was seeded first, in the opening round. She was very nice to me, very nice, and even tried to give me a game, but I was so terrified I just froze."

Once the tennis ended, she reluctantly turned to running. Lois calls it a "godsend."

"I'd always run a bit, mostly on days when I'd get rained out of playing tennis," she said. "I'd never done more than four or five miles until then, even though I'd always envied people who run the marathon.

"Today I've run six New York Marathons. My first was in 1987, the year my husband died. Unfortunately, I didn't pay attention up in the Bronx and tripped and fell and just couldn't finish. But I've finished every year since.

"I've only run the New York Marathons. My son Johnny says the Boston is quite tough. New York is pretty level. I've always been very slow but it doesn't matter in certain age groups! There's just no one else left! As a result, I've gotten a few prizes. I'm doing well now that I'm in the 80-plus bracket, but in a couple of years there will be a few others right on my heels. So I'll probably have to wait until I hit 90 to win some more."

Lois' memories of the six marathons range from exquisite street scenes, little human dramas encountered along the way, to the adrenaline rush of standing—along with 25,000 other equally nervous people—at the starting gate, waiting for the starter's gun. ("You just can't believe how exciting it all is!")

Two months after her first marathon, Lois walked into her neighborhood grocery store. When she brought her groceries to the checkout counter, she found the clerks laughing and pointing.

"When I asked them why, they showed me the current *National Enquirer*," she said. "Sure enough, in an issue with Liberace on the cover, there was a story about the 'three gutsy grandmas' who ran the New York. That was the year I fell, but they told how I 'bravely limped home, but was all set to do it again the next year.' I never talked to them, but that was almost exactly what had happened, so they must have called the Roadrunners for the story."

Still, 1989 might have been her last marathon if it hadn't been for Dick Traum and the Achilles group.

"Dick Traum lost one of his legs in an accident in his 20s," Lois said. "Years later, he became the first amputee to run the New York Marathon. He founded the Achilles Track Club, which he named because each person has some weakness. Since then he has gone all over the world, founding chapters in China, Russia, Poland, everywhere.

"Anyway, I discovered these people and it is just so very inspiring. There must be 100 members of that group who run in the New York Marathon. There's one woman who has multiple sclerosis and takes 24 hours—but she completes it. Anyway, since then I've run as a volunteer with them. They're all so inspiring, so bright, so funny, that they've kept me running.

"I don't think I would have gone on with it without them."

At the same time, running has its own rewards, Lois said.

"There's really nothing spiritual about what I do or why, except the wonderful highs you get after it," she said. "For a month after a marathon, you're on top of the world."

If Lois isn't the typical marathoner, she doesn't prepare for marathons in a typical way, either.

For instance: "I wake up very early each morning, full of energy. I have to run in the morning, otherwise I'm hopeless— I just can't do it. I greatly admire these people who work all day, then come home and run."

Or: "You know that people who run like to eat pasta, but I hate pasta, so I don't eat it before I run a marathon. I'll eat granola and things like that instead."

Actually, her diet is basically unchanged from before her marathon-running days.

"I eat a lot of yogurt; I'm practically a vegetarian," she said. "Of course, in my long-lived family, my father hated vegetables and ate virtually only meat. It seems to me that the meat is not as good as it used to be, either. So while I'll eat some chicken, mostly I eat lots of vegetables and fruit. I notice I'm not as hungry when I exercise.

"I used to eat a lot of meat, about a pound a day, but I switched about 10 years ago when it got so expensive and all of these terrible articles came out about it. I've done just fine without it."

Nor have her vices—or lack of them—changed all that much in recent years.

"I've never smoked, except at boarding school when I wasn't supposed to," Lois said. "I quit when I had a boyfriend tell me I didn't look as sophisticated as I thought I did. He bullied me to quit. None of the rest of my family ever smoked.

"I used to like to drink a little, but now it gives me a headache. But even then I only liked a little shot of Jack Daniels. I've always had a very light head, so I couldn't ever drink much."

The end result of a sensible diet and a good gene pool? Lois had never had any major health problems—until early in 1992.

"Just after the marathon, I was diagnosed as needing a hysterectomy," she said. "They found a malignant cancer and I received radiation treatment for it. Apparently, the doctors got most of it. I was able to resume running during the radiation treatment, so it hasn't set me back all that much.

"Other than that, I've never been sick, which is very annoying to some people. I've always had good doctors, whom I loved seeing, and they've all been very supportive of my running. They've said, 'Do anything you feel like doing.' It makes so much sense, and they say the same things to a lot of the people in the Achilles group. If you keep on running, you don't have time to think about yourself."

Lois' calm, even-keeled demeanor also may have had something to do with her continued steady recovery from the surgery.

"When I was diagnosed with cancer, I was pretty fatalistic

about it," she said. "Either I made it or I didn't, but I wasn't worried. I'll run as long as I feel well, and I feel no different now than I did before the surgery.

"I'm mostly an optimistic person, although twice a year I go into a depression. It is the most extraordinary thing. It happens every spring and fall and I know it is coming and try to fight it off. I just love the summer, and when it really gets cold I'm back on track again. This has gone on ever since my husband died.

"Finally, my doctor prescribed Prozac for me—and I've heard some perfectly dreadful things about Prozac since—but it clears it up."

Lois said that she almost always runs with young people, partly because there are few people in her age bracket who continue to run competitively. Not that she minds. Lois said she believes it's a good idea to be with younger people.

"My husband and I joined an amateur Gilbert and Sullivan group years ago and I've stayed active in it ever since," she said. "I've worked in all the shows, never on stage, but I prompt or help with the tickets, and go to the parties. It's always with younger people. It's different when you have an interest in common other than just going out with younger people to be with younger people. They call me their 'Ann Landers' and tell me all of their love problems—you need a score card to keep up with them!"

Not surprisingly, some of that advice involves fitness and health matters as well.

"My advice to a younger person who wants to still be running at age 81 is that you can't stop and start," she said, "you've got to keep right at it. I need more exercise now than before. After my operation, I wasn't allowed to run for a while and it was very hard to get back. I ran 10 miles two weeks ago and it took forever, but I was determined to finish. But if you have your health and feel like it, there's nothing like it.

"Now for a senior who has not been active, I'd suggest that they talk to their doctor, then work up to it. Start slowly. I encourage other seniors to run and there are a surprising number of them who do run regularly. I think there are fifteen 70-year-olds who run in the marathon each year. And it goes all of the way up to a 94-year-old who comes over from Germany every year.

"I know of one 70-year-old man whose family tried to put him in a nursing home. He was furious and, unbeknownst to

them, began exercising. He's in his 80s and he's showing no
signs of being forced into a nursing home now."

Nor does Lois Schieffelin appear to be ready for a rocking
chair any time soon. Not only did she run her fastest marathon
in 1991, but it was the beginning of an extended brush with
fame for the genial New Yorker.

"Two days after the marathon, my telephone rang," she
said. "I thought it was a friend playing a joke on me because
she said she was calling from 'The David Letterman Show.' But
it was no joke. The gal who called was very nice and she
interviewed me over the phone about the marathon, then
asked if I was interested in appearing on Letterman the following
night, which was November 7, 1991, and I said, 'You bet
I would!'

"Of course, there was this great headline the next day in
The New York Post about Letterman fighting with NBC over
who would replace Johnny Carson. The headline said, 'NBC
You Later.' And all of my friends said, 'See there, you've finished
off Letterman!'"

But Lois reports that no matter what his problems off-camera,
Letterman was a perfect gentleman during the show.

"I didn't meet him until I got onstage," she said. "I was on
for about five minutes. I came on last and he kept talking
about an 80-year-old woman running a marathon and how
amazing it was. He said, 'You could fly to California in
that time!'

"I'd never watched Letterman before, so I didn't know what
to expect. He kept making a big thing about ordering clams for
the whole studio audience and finally, just before he ran out
of time, he had clams brought in. He offered me a clam, but I
hate clams and told him so. He seemed to be somewhat taken
aback by that.

"Since then, I've watched him several times and I think he
would have been better replacing Johnny than Jay Leno. Don't
you think so?"

But even 15 minutes worth of fame—or five minutes, as in
Lois' case—can have its drawbacks as well. Lois said she "got
very full" of herself following the *Letterman* appearance and a
subsequent news feature on ABC.

"Shortly after that, I stopped on my daily run to get a salad
at a wonderful place," she said. "I was in my running outfit,
helping myself to salad when this nice-looking man came up
and said, 'Good morning, jogger.'

"I said, 'How did you know I was a runner?' thinking he'd seen me before on TV.

"He said, 'Anybody who would go out in the street dressed like that *has* to be a jogger—or crazy!'

"By the time I recovered my wits, he was gone. I keep going by that deli, hoping to catch him there again!"

What's ahead for Lois Schieffelin? She'd like to keep running, do more marathons, stay fit and active for the foreseeable future. And she likes her age just the way it is.

"Forty was my worst birthday," she said. "I thought that's when you get to the end. But you change as you go on. I have as much fun now as I had then. I'm quite a showoff and people make much more of you at 80 running the marathon than they do when you're 50. At 80 you can be peculiar and say strange things and can get away with so much more!"

Chapter 18

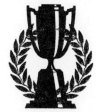

Dr. Eugene Shirk

READING, PENNSYLVANIA—His real name is Dr. Eugene L. Shirk, but everybody calls him "Coach." Except, of course, those who call him "Sir." Gene Shirk is 91—the oldest college coach in any sport in America. Maybe the oldest coach of *any* kind.

But he's no figurehead. Gene coaches, travels, even eats with the men's cross-country team at Albright College, near Reading. In 1992, the team had its best record ever with an impressive 11–2 record.

As a result, in recent years Albright has been the host for CNN, ESPN, *The Philadelphia Inquirer, Sports Illustrated*—literally dozens of newspapers, magazines, and television programs—as they've all sought to learn something about the man who truly deserves to be called a college "senior."

What the cameras and reporters have found is a delightful gentleman who looks 30 years younger. He is trim and spry, and has a Pennsylvania Dutch accent as thick as homemade apple cider. His athletes are obviously crazy about him, but coaching is only part of the Gene Shirk story.

Gene was born in Adamstown, a small town in Pennsylvania, on April 14, 1901, about 10 miles from Reading. Save for a stint at college and his term in the service, Gene has *never* lived more than 10 miles from Reading. Adamstown was too small to have its own high school, so Gene took the trolley each day to high school in Ephrata, Pennsylvania, about half an hour away.

Following his graduation, Gene went to work as a silk weaver in Reading, since his family could not afford a college education for him. After a year, however, he began to attend the Franklin & Marshall College in Lancaster, Pennsylvania, where he was a Phi Beta Kappa graduate in 1924.

"I wanted to become a lawyer, but didn't have the money to go on to law school, and there was no money for scholarships at that time, so I decided to teach for two years—and then go to law school," Gene said.

"Late in the summer, I found a job at Birdsboro High School, which is also about 10 miles from Reading. I accepted a position there teaching math in the four upper grades, and coaching basketball and track.

"They offered me $1,300 to teach. My college professor said, 'Don't take this job unless they pay you $1,400.' But the Birdsboro principal said, 'I'm only allowed $1,300. The school board won't let me pay any more than that. But I'll tell you what I'm going to do. If you do a good job, I'll give you a $100 bonus. And I want to tell you that I got my bonus."

Gene liked teaching and coaching so much that, when his self-imposed two years had elapsed, he decided he wasn't going to go to law school after all.

"Luckily, I inherited some very fine boys. Because I hadn't played much basketball, he said, the first thing I did was buy a book on basketball! Fortunately, the boys and I had a good time, so they thought I was a good coach. Also, I had some very good students in math, so I kept on teaching and coaching for 18 years.

"I ended up as principal and then we started baseball and cross-country as well. Sometimes I had to coach both the boys and the girls. In track, I had to coach boys and girls, as well as senior- and junior-high students for the first two years."

Gene's successes at Birdsboro caught the eye of other schools, including nearby Albright College. But he refused all offers until 1942, when he accepted the position of athletic director at Albright—but only under the condition that he be allowed to continue to coach track and teach a few math classes.

"But no more had I arrived at Albright on July 1, 1942, than I was inducted into the service for World War II on the 5th," he said. "I spent three years and one month in the service as a meteorologist in the Air Corps."

After the war, the position at Albright College was still waiting and Gene happily settled down for a long career in academe.

"Then in 1963, I was approached to run for mayor of Reading," he said. "Reading was very corrupt then and I didn't want to. But people kept asking me to run for the job, and eventually I said I would. I was probably the most naive man ever elected! I left Albright—although I had to teach my classes for a few more weeks because the semester wasn't quite over and I wanted to teach to the end. I became mayor and served for four years."

As is his custom, Gene understated the difficulties he faced in Reading. It had the reputation of being one of the most corrupt cities in America at the time, and it was only through his firm leadership—with an assist from Robert Kennedy and various federal operatives—that the city was eventually cleaned up.

After four exhausting but rewarding years, Gene served as the assistant to the president of Albright for four years.

"Then they were after me to run again, and, of course, my wife says I never say 'no,'" Gene said. "So, I said I would. But at that time, there were no real difficulties so far as crime and corruption in the city. And since Reading is definitely a Democratic community with about three Democrats to one Republican, the only time a Republican has a chance is if there is something going on to make the people desperate. This time there was nothing like that, so no one thought I could win.

"But my campaign manager took me around, and we went door-to-door. Even the newspaper didn't think we could win. But we surprised everybody. I was the only Republican in City Hall for four years."

During Gene's second term as mayor, New York University received a grant from the National Science Foundation to investigate whether two-way television would be of any benefit to senior citizens. The NYU researchers chose Reading for the pilot program because of its involvement with seniors and its progressive cable television franchise, Berks Cable.

"They came to see me in City Hall and asked if we would help," Gene said. "I said, 'Only if it doesn't cost us anything.' We went in it with them and eventually they won the grant. It was supposed to be an 18-month affair."

In short order, the new two-way technology hooked up several senior centers and hundreds of homes in Reading. Senior citizens became actively involved in the management, production, and talent in the daily telecasts. When the 18 months were up, the City of Reading asked to keep the expensive equipment to continue the unique public-access programming.

"So they told a group of us that they would give us the equipment for one dollar *if* we would continue to run the program," Gene said. "We had no money and we didn't realize at that time how much it cost to operate. So we formed a non-profit organization and tried it."

The next step was to elect Gene as director/president of the organization. In short order, he began raising the money to keep it broadcasting indefinitely.

"It wasn't until then that I realized how wonderful it was and how much it helped senior citizens," he said. "Seniors who had sat home doing nothing now came out and became producers, MCs of programs, even technical people. Most of them were amateurs who had never done anything like this before. But now they were designing and producing programs. Many of the shows had people calling in, or they'd see someone in another studio. By that time it had expanded until it covered the entire cable system. It was then an open affair.

"At the same time, they asked me to do a one-hour program with high school students called *Bridging the Generation Gap*. I didn't want to do it. I said, 'I'm too old to deal with young people like that.' But they insisted I try it and I did. That was 17 years ago and I'm still doing it every Friday morning! It's another two-way thing. The young people are in their studio and I'm in my studio. And when they come on, I ask them what they want to talk about and we talk about it. And home viewers call in, too. We see each other on a split screen. It has gotten to be quite interesting, quite challenging."

Reading's two-way, public-access system remains one of the premier programs of its kind in the world. Producers and politicians from Germany to Japan and all 50 states have come to Reading to study it.

Incidentally, the original by-laws of the new non-profit organization specifically mandated that no officer could hold his or her post more than three years. When Gene's time as president was up, they simply changed the by-laws.

"Today we have our very lovely studio, have a budget of close to $300,000 a year, and we're growing," he said.

In 1976, the athletic director who had succeeded Gene at Albright asked him to return and coach once again.

"I said, 'Oh no, I'm too old to get back into coaching.' But he said, 'But we really need somebody.' My wife and I live close to the campus and I said, 'Since you're the one asking me and we've been such good friends, I'll try it.'

"So now I'm still coaching, still coaching men's cross-country. And that's how I got all of this publicity."

Through half a century of coaching, hundreds of races, and

tens of thousands of people, Gene has an incredible storehouse of memories. So many, in fact, that he's hesitant to single *any* out as the most memorable, for fear of slighting a hundred more just as outstanding.

He will talk about a letter he received just days ago from a former student whom he once counseled to stay in school. The student ultimately became head of a department at the University of West Virginia.

"I didn't remember that talk, of course," Gene said, "but the letter went on giving me so much credit. I don't think I did anything—except to talk to him and try to talk him into realizing that you need an education. And he never forgot that. Those are things that mean a great deal to me."

Gene claims to have trouble remembering any of his accomplishments as a coach, but will quickly talk about a poor student from a tiny town who came from a virtually illiterate family—but who eventually became a member of both the Albright Hall of Fame and the faculty at Temple University.

"I think about him once in a while," Gene said. "It seems like you're more likely to remember outstanding individuals that you had. But when you coach so many, you could think of a thousand."

For Gene, the student athletes are what keep him coming to the track year after year.

Cross-country practice starts a few days before the fall semester begins. Most of the team arrives then for two-a-day workouts that continue until classes begin.

"After school starts, we try to get together at 3:30 p.m.," Gene said. "Some days it's a long run, even up to 12 miles. Other days, it is a short distance, a short workout to work on speed. We alternate distance and speed. I have a good assistant, Don Gottshall, who used to be my captain when I was coaching here at Albright. He plans the sessions. He's good at it, he knows what I like.

"I am not as gung-ho to win as Don is; he wants to win. I guess that makes for the good combination you need. We want that desire to win, but it shouldn't be the all-important reason for running. I want them to enjoy running. If they're not, then I really don't think they should be doing it.

"We try to keep them happy by doing things they enjoy. I vary the program so that they're not running at the same place all of the time. We go round to different parts of the city and county around here, different parks and places like that to vary the places to run.

"We like to win; I think you ought to learn to win. But the important thing is for you to reach your optimum. It is up to us to try and help them reach that goal. Whether they are last in a meet or first, it is improvement that is important."

Gene accompanies the team every Saturday during the eight-week cross-country season and, for those who qualify, through the Division III qualifying meets.

"If the men and women's teams go together, we go on a bus," he said. "If not, the men or women go in a van.

"We are fortunate to be in an area where there are so many colleges within 20, 30, 40, or 50 miles. So we very seldom stop for a meal anywhere. In cross-country, runners have to be careful when they eat. So we all eat breakfast together before we go. If we run in the morning, we take sack lunches along and eat on the way back. But we usually get home in time to see the tail end of the football game. Very seldom do we get back after dark."

The Middle Atlantic Conference is made up of small, liberal arts schools. There are a number of such schools in eastern Pennsylvania, with a few in New Jersey and in Maryland—Moravian, Gettysberg, Muhlenberg, Delaware Valley, Juniata and the others—all within 50 miles of Albright.

"This schedule is only in the fall of the year," Gene said. "I'm not with them the rest of the year. They come to the house once in a while because our house is not far from campus.

"I eat with them in the evening when I can. Monday night I bowl, Tuesday I play tennis. Ordinarily, I like to eat the evening meal with the team where we all sit together.

My wife is always glad when the season is over because I eat with her more at nights during the off-season. The only thing that changes for me is that I don't go up to Albright every afternoon. I do go up sometimes and have coffee with the athletic director, who is also retired, and some other people. I am on the campus a lot, but I have nothing to do officially except in the fall."

Don't believe it. Gene Shirk *always* has plenty to do. He says that is a factor in keeping him young. Gene attributes his longevity to several factors: genetics, exercise, diet, and an inquisitive, passionate outlook on life.

As for the genetics part, he has a brother and a sister who both lived past 100.

"I don't act my age," Gene said. "But I know a lot of it is that I had good parents—with good genes."

As for exercise, Gene believes in moderation in all things.

"I don't have a fetish for exercise, per se," he said. "I believe in being fit. I don't think you should go into exercise just for the sake of it. Take weight lifting. If you want to build up your body, that's fine. If you want to walk for exercise, that's fine. My philosophy is that you keep fit by doing what you enjoy doing.

"For example, my wife Annadora loves to swim. She enjoys going to the Y and swimming half a mile at least twice a week while I'm off playing tennis. I play tennis and golf and bowl, and she swims. I think you should do the things you enjoy and keep fit that way. Don't do something if you don't enjoy it. If you run or walk just because you want to keep fit, *that's* not enjoying life. I think you should be doing the things you like to do."

As for diet, Gene again gives much of the credit to his parents.

"I come from a family that never needed to worry about our weight," he said. "We were always skinny and eating never bothered us. So I eat anything. Being a Pennsylvania Dutchman, I love Pennsylvania Dutch cooking. I love meat, potatoes, and vegetables.

"It depends on the individual, but it is probably better for you not to eat a lot of meat. I'm not a great meat eater. I like a small portion of meat. I love chicken. Really, when I order out anywhere, it is usually seafood. I don't order meat because the portions are too large.

"Now, I do love desserts. I want you to know my wife makes great desserts. And in my cereal each morning, I use half and half. I couldn't enjoy my cereal without half and half. I love soups. For a meal, maybe I'll have a glass of wine, a bowl of soup and dessert. If I make soup at home out of the can, I use half and half. If I have one bad habit, it is maybe desserts. And half and half."

Well, one bad habit in 91 years isn't too bad.

The last element in Gene Shirk's recipe for a long and happy life involves the mind. Or, more precisely, the active use of the mind. Gene works it out as vigorously as any other muscle.

In addition to his two-way cable-access show, he also hosts a national issues-oriented program founded by the Kettering Foundation. The show makes use of the two-way cable hookup to conduct an on-the-spot viewer polls.

"I just finished one that didn't make me happy because it was three Tuesday nights in succession," Gene said, "which meant I couldn't play tennis. Now that that's over, I'm back.

"I drop into the studio almost every day. There are checks to sign or things to do. We also have monthly board meetings.

"But the one thing that has helped me is that television program I do on Friday mornings, *Bridging the Generation Gap*. It keeps me in touch with the young people. If you're going to enjoy life, you must like people of all ages. You must meet with them—you can't sit home. I think one of the worst things senior citizens do is sit at home and not get out and do things."

Does it sound like Gene is an optimist? Believe it. He's also unfailingly good-natured, something of a wit, and deeply religious. The lifelong Methodist says that he is a firm believer in the power of prayer.

"No matter what you call it, I still think if you really work hard at something and believe in it, you can do it," he said. "I should qualify that. I don't believe that, if you ask for personal things, you can expect to get them. But I'm a strong believer in prayer and even meditation.

"Cross-country runners—almost everyone that likes to run—wants about 10 minutes on their own to prepare before a race, to get ready for the race. I think some pray, some meditate, and some concentrate on just how they are going to run. They get worked up into the running spirit. I firmly believe that you must concentrate, whether you call it prayer or not. I do."

There's not a whole lot left for Gene to do. They've named the football stadium/track field after him at Albright. He's been athletic director and he's been mayor. He still has his own television show—two, in fact. He's achieved a measure of fame through the national media. His teams have won and his teams have lost. Now his life revolves around his family, cross-country, and his faith.

"I have no ambitions for anything particular that I still want to do," he said. "My whole lifetime, things have seemed to happen and I don't know why. I was asked to run for mayor and I have no idea why they picked me. I go to meetings, I keep quiet, I don't open my mouth—next thing I know, I've been elected president. It is things like that, that have happened.

"I don't really have any big plans for the future—in any way, shape, or form. If my wife wants to take a trip, we'll go. I believe this very strongly: don't live in the past. I enjoy today.

"But most important is my family. I strongly believe that

people must love others if they want to enjoy living. All ages, young and old, all sorts of people, from all walks of life."

Gene was 53 when his last daughter was born. He has a granddaughter who isn't three yet. (His son Bill was a star cross-country performer for Albright in the mid-1950s.)

"Bill's daughters are older, so I don't see that much of them," Gene said. "But the younger ones live only three hours away, and we see them as much as we possibly can. And they just love me—they call me 'DeeDa'—and I just love them. I could spend days with them and never get tired of being with the kids. And for some reason, they enjoy being with me, too. If you really put yourself on their level, they know that you're concentrating on them, playing with them, reading to them— they just learn to love you for that.

"I think too many adults, if they go visit a family, spend all their time talking with the other adults while the poor children don't get much attention. They love them, but they don't spend that much time with them. I spend my time with the grandchildren and let the adults talk!"

And so the days go with Eugene L. Shirk. He's been to nine Olympic Games, has seen Jessie Owens and Adolph Hitler, yet prefers to talk about taking his 11-year-old grandson to Atlanta in 1996. One morning he's swapping one-liners with a feisty ninth grader on *Bridging the Generation Gap*. That afternoon he's standing at the base of Mount Penn, timing his boys as they return from their daily run. That evening is spent romping on the floor with the grandkids and wondering if there's any half and half left in the fridge for a late-night snack. Days continue to flow in a gentle, autumnal cycle, each one fresh and rewarding—but as comfortable as an old slipper.

"I just don't believe in living in the past," he said reflectively. "I think about today and hope for tomorrow! Hope that I can see my grandchildren tomorrow.

"There is one thing I feel very strongly about. I like to talk to senior citizens. I like to make them—especially those who haven't quite retired yet—realize that you retire *to* something and not *from* something. You must have something to do.

"People can enjoy life. I don't believe in worrying, and I don't believe in losing your temper, because you're the only one that suffers from it! Things like that are important. You've got to love people at all levels and all ages. I think the one reason I've been fortunate is that I inherited that sort of disposition. My parents didn't get all worked up about things.

I didn't go to bed at night worrying about something. If I couldn't do anything that night, I'd wait until the next morning. And I feel very strongly about that: you can't worry about what's *going* to happen. Wait and *see* what's going to happen.

"That's something of my philosophy when I talk to senior citizens in particular. If you want to enjoy life, don't live in the past. Think about the future."

Chapter 19

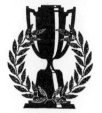

Esther Slager

SUN CITY WEST, ARIZONA—Rhythm Tappers line captain, Esther Slager, is busy putting her girls through a rigorous rehearsal. The group is going to perform next week at the Sundome and she's concerned the enthusiasm isn't what it should be.

When it comes time for Esther to practice one of her solos, she turns to the choreographer and says, "Gee, you know, I'm a little tired today." Her New York accent is untouched by her years in this ritzy desert retirement community.

The choreographer only laughs.

"Esther, I don't worry about you," he says. "When you get on that stage, you light it up!"

It's true. The 69-year-old pride of Yonkers, New York, still has the looks and gams that prompted war-weary grunts and swabbies to name her the USO's "Miss Foxhole of 1942" (the girl they'd most like to get caught in a fox hole with)!

Esther is a bundle of energy, with a dazzling smile. She is wearing black sequins, and a flashing, sparkling pin that says, "5,6,7,8." (Tap dancing, Esther patiently explains, *always* begins at the count of eight.)

After rehearsal, she cheerfully admits to being born in 1923. Age is obviously not an issue in Sun City West, where the average age is 62.

"I began tap dance at age nine in a local dance studio," she said. "I took lessons at the local studio almost until the beginning of the war. I wanted to go to dancing lessons earlier, but I don't think my mother could afford them at that time. She said, 'No, I can't do it right now.' So I used to dance in the street. My mother's friends said, 'You should give that child dance lessons.' And that's when it started.

"When I was about 16 and still going to school, I wanted to audition on Broadway. But my mother wouldn't let me go. 'No show business,' she said."

After high school, Esther took lessons from the well-known choreographer, Ernest Carlos. Soon she was dancing professionally in New York and on Long Island. Still, she was surprised when her mother allowed her to join a USO troupe after the war broke out.

"I traveled with them, entertaining at Army camps, stage-door canteens, and some Naval bases," she said. "I traveled with the USO up and down the East Coast. The group did go overseas, but my mom wouldn't allow me to go with them. I was just 17 and she said, 'No way!' I met a lot of nice sailors and soldiers, though."

After the war, Esther met Mr. Slager, and the couple quickly got married and settled in Yonkers. But the pressure of helping with the family business and raising their children meant that she put her tap shoes away.

"We took time out to raise our two boys: Michael, who is an emergency-room physician in Boston; and Richard, who has a limo service in New York," she said. "And I have two grandchildren, Jeremy and Jonathan.

"I did not resume dancing until we moved to Sun City in 1983 when we retired. I learned of the Rhythm Tappers here and I immediately joined the group. There were only about 40 of us at that time. Since then, I've performed in all their variety shows—nine of them and counting, mostly at the Sundome, which holds about 7,000 people."

There is no age limit for the Rhythm Tappers, but there is a waiting list. Esther said a number of applicants want to join just for the exercise the group's strenuous rehearsals provide.

"They don't want to do the shows, or they are not capable, or whatever," she said. "They just enjoy it.

"We practice three times a week, Mondays, Wednesdays, and Saturdays, by groups or classes. We have the beginners that start at 7 a.m. in the morning and each class lasts one hour. The other classes are at 8, 8:30, 9, 10—and I'm the teacher's assistant in the advanced class at 11 o'clock. That's the most advanced."

In 1986, her husband was killed in a traffic accident. A woman ran a stop sign and hit him while he was riding on his motorcycle. The tragedy shook Esther, who threw herself even more into the Rhythm Tappers.

"In 1988, I was voted the president of the Rhythm Tappers club," she said. "By then we had maybe 100 members. Now in 1992, we have 180 members.

"From the beginning, I've been putting programs together for the Rhythm Tappers and directing the road shows. We perform mostly in different places in Arizona: Tuscon, Scottsdale, Mesa. Also, we do some charity work, performing in nursing homes and hospitals."

In addition to regular performances at their small theater in Sun City West—which Esther often programs and directs—the Rhythm Tappers frequently perform in the nearby Sundome.

"I do a lot of solos in the shows, and the Rhythm Tappers come in and do numbers—and that's always fun," she said. "We learn different routines to tap. Not all of us are in the big shows, but we do standard Broadway-style musicals. I just enjoy entertaining people."

Under Esther's energetic tutelage, the Rhythm Tappers have begun to receive national attention as well. They've been featured in a number of newspaper and magazine articles and were once spotlighted in a PBS program on senior health and fitness.

"We've also been performing overseas every year for the past few years," Esther said. "The first year, 1989, we went to Japan on a cultural exchange and we danced with the people over there. That was very interesting because we lived with the Japanese people in their homes. We didn't stay in hotels.

"In 1990, we went to Russia. We left Russia just before the coup—we didn't have any idea anything was happening until we stopped in Copenhagen on the way home. In Russia we performed in some beautiful theaters, but I don't remember any of the names. This past year, 1991, we were in Australia. We danced there and that was quite interesting. And now we're working on Europe."

Not, of course, that Esther is consumed with dancing and the Rhythm Tappers. Like the majority of Sun City West residents, she's an active volunteer for charity.

"I do take time out to volunteer at the local hospital and that keeps me busy," she said. "I like to keep fit. I golf, bowl, and bicycle ride. I play bridge, mah-jongg, and canasta.

"I also belong to another group composed of older dancing gals. A gentleman came out here and said he was from Hollywood and what have you. He called one day, found out about me, and I joined. And we've gone to Las Vegas and we did dance at the Sahara Hotel as the Christopher Girls. It is not so much tap dancing, it's a little different. I find that I'm too busy with Rhythm Tappers, so I've shied away from it a little bit. It was mostly show dance. He had some show girls in it, mostly jazz, and things like that.

"So I really keep busy. I exercise and dance three–four times a week. I think it is important."

Esther's also conscious of the benefits of a healthy diet.

"I eat sensibly and I take my vitamins," she said. "I'm not a vegetarian; I do eat lean red meat occasionally—but I can go without meat for sometimes three months. I do watch my weight.

"I came to Sun City in good health. My doctors are very supportive. Every time I go to my doctor for a checkup, he says, 'You're in great shape for a woman of your age—114 pounds.'"

It doesn't take but a few minutes with Esther Slager and her infectious laugh to know that this is a positive, optimistic lady.

"I guess I just look at the good side of people," she said. "I try to be kind. You know, it is so much easier to be nice. I try to help others who are less fortunate—I feel like I'm blowing my own horn here.

"But you need to enjoy what you do. The main thing is to keep busy and help others. You know that saying, 'Do unto others as you would have them do unto you?' I'm looking forward to a long and healthy life."

Does age matter at all to a person's physical fitness? Esther says "No!"

"I think young, I think positive," she said. "I can do most anything a younger person can do because I am in shape. Dancing really helps, I'm telling you.

"If I didn't do what I do, I'd probably have a lot more weight, and probably wouldn't be as healthy. I tell older people to get in there, start exercising, eat sensibly—and by all means, join the Rhythm Tappers! It is never too late.

"In the Rhythm Tappers, we had one lady who was 83, and we have a lot of people in their 70s: Age doesn't matter. You can take control of your life at 65 or above. It is *never* too late."

Strangely enough, that's the same advice she gives young people who want to be dancing to Gershwin and Cole Porter tunes at age 69:

"Watch what you eat, get a lot of exercise, and I would tell them—dance! Join the Rhythm Tappers! That's about it."

Clearly, Esther's passion is still dance. She says she can't remember a time when it wasn't.

"I love music, but I don't how I could explain it," she said, "it's just in my blood. It's just so exciting.

"I've always had that, wanting to get up and do it. When I was a little girl—and I started kind of late, actually, since 9 years old is not early for a dancer—I used to watch people dancing anywhere I could.

"I had a dentist once whose wife was a dancer—but by then she was teaching dancing. He said, 'You know, Esther, I would sponsor you if you would just let me.' And I woulda, if it had been left up to me. But my mother, she just wouldn't allow it.

"If I had had the chance to audition for Broadway, I think my life would have been a little different. That was my highest goal in those days—that was about it. Well, also in those days they had musicals out in Hollywood with people like Ann Miller and Esther Williams and I used to think about that a lot. But I wasn't allowed to do it."

But nothing can keep the irrepressible Esther Slager dwelling on the past for long.

"At this stage, in dancing, I don't expect to go to Hollywood and be a star or anything like that," she said. "But it's great now, it really is.

"I was once asked to dance in Phoenix. It was one other person and myself and we did a number titled 'Sing, Sing, Sing' and when we finished, I noticed Ann Miller was there. She lives out in Sedonia, AZ. Afterwards, she came over to us. She said she thought we were wonderful and really praised us. That was a *real* highlight."

Chapter 20

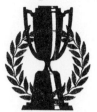

Dr. Paul Spangler

SAN LUIS OBISPO, CALIFORNIA—If you happen to be up at, say, 4:30 a.m. any Tuesday, Thursday, or Saturday morning in this sleepy California town, you might see 93-year-old Dr. Paul Spangler padding silently through the quiet streets. After his seven-mile run, he'll swim a half-mile at the town pool.

After swimming, he'll take a moment to fuss about his "miserable" performance in the 1991 New York City Marathon—26.2 miles in just under nine hours.

"I'm too damned old," he'll mutter. "And I went out too fast."

Well, he probably *did* get out of the blocks too fast. It's not hard to do when you get swept up by a crowd of 24,000 runners. But too old? The man who has held 200 running records in his lifetime, *all* since the age of 70? The man who, at age 79, once ran a 3 hour, 59 minute marathon? The same man who every Monday, Wednesday, and Friday morning works out with weights?

Too old? Not a chance.

Dr. Paul Spangler has become one of the premier runners in the world ("Well, I've outlived everybody else," he grumbles), and a tireless advocate of exercise and sensible eating. His story has been detailed in newspapers and magazines ranging from *The New York Times* to the *Los Angeles Times*.

But it wasn't always that way. There was a time when he weighed more than 215 pounds, ate a fatty diet, and lead a sedentary life.

Today he works out daily, eats right and weighs 130 pounds.

"I shrank," he said simply.

Paul was born March 18, 1899. His father—who lived to be 85—played a little bare-handed baseball, and his mother rowed crew at Wellesey, but they are the only athletes in his background.

Paul's own athletic career in high school and college was equally undistinguished. After graduating from the University of Oregon, he attended Harvard Medical School, where he was one of three *magna cum laude* graduates ("I've outlived the other two") in 1923.

Although he dreamed of becoming a medical missionary (his father was a minister), Paul eventually settled into private practice in Portland, Oregon, where he and his wife began a family that would eventually include four children.

After war erupted in Europe, Paul, a medical reserve officer, was called up to active duty in April 1941. He was assigned to the Naval Hospital at Pearl Harbor where he was serving as acting chief of surgery at the hospital on December 7, 1941.

"At the time of the attack, my wife and daughter were just getting ready to go on a picnic at Barber's Point," he recalled. "Before we left, I got a call from the hospital, telling me that all hell had broken loose. When I got out there, the chief of surgery met me at the door and said, 'You've got to take over, I'm busy here.'

"I was the first surgeon to operate on the first American casualty of World War II. There's no question about that. They brought in a civilian who had been wounded in the Pacific around Midway Island somewhere. The Navy flew him in and he was the first casualty we received. His leg was shattered around the ankle, it was completely destroyed, and he needed an amputation. That was the first classical amputation that was done—and the only classical surgery. Beyond that was just emergency dressing of wounds and sending them over to the mainland."

Paul was a member of a team of four doctors who worked non-stop for the next 72 hours. Since the Naval Hospital had only two operating rooms, doctors operated for two hours and then were off two hours doing pre-ops on the incoming wounded.

After Pearl Harbor, Paul was selected to oversee construction of additional hospitals in Hawaii by the Seabees, as well as serve as executive officer and chief of surgery.

"Finally, I had my belly full of Naval construction," he said, "and eventually the Navy sent me back to Brooklyn, New York, to get the USS hospital ship *Repose* manned and supplied for the upcoming invasion of Japan."

The war ended before the *Repose* could reach Japan, and

Paul returned to civilian life. But after Pearl Harbor, life in private practice in Portland left much to be desired.

"The doctors who had not been called to active duty had all bought apartment houses and farms while I was in the Navy," Paul told the *Los Angeles Times*. "They controlled the hospitals. We were nothing."

Disillusioned, Paul re-entered the Navy, this time as a captain. Before he retired in 1959, he'd realized his childhood dream of being a medical missionary by serving aboard the first hospital ship sent by Project Hope to Southeast Asia.

Back in the United States, Paul visited the California Men's Colony at San Luis Obispo to visit an old Navy friend. By the end of the day he'd signed on as a surgeon at the prison.

"In Portland, I belonged to the athletic club and I got a little exercise, but nothing regular or purposeful," he said. "Nothing I'd call real training—and nothing like I have done for the last 25 years.

"I started running when I was 67. I didn't retire from medical practice until 1969 when I was 69. In this state you have to retire at age 70. By then I had been running for two years, mostly to get my weight down."

But, as he told *The New York Times*, he had another reason for running. Coronary disease was killing too many people he cared about.

"Friends, relatives, peers, classmates; they were all dying. I had no indication of any trouble, but I began to get a fear of developing heart disease. I knew there was a better way to live, and I knew it was about time I did something about it."

After Paul's retirement, a track coach from Southern California came up to San Luis Obispo to organize a masters track meet. It was the first Paul had heard of such a thing.

"So I thought, 'Gee, I guess I'll see what this is all about,'" he said. "So at 10 a.m., I ran in the mile, and then came back home to work on an exercise station which we were building for a fitness trail to put in one of the city parks.

"Then I went back after lunch to run the three-mile race. People started coming up and pounding me on the back and I asked, 'What's all of this for?' And they said, 'Well, you set a new world record for your age in the mile!' So I said, 'What are the records for two miles and three miles in my age bracket?' They looked those up and told me, and I predicted I could knock three minutes off the two-mile, and five minutes off the three-mile race!

"At the end of the day I'd set three new world records in my age bracket in the first track meet I'd ever entered!

"For a fellow who had been a failure in track and baseball in high school and college, that was quite stimulating! So naturally I've been hooked on competition ever since."

Paul has set a host of records—he estimates as many as 200—since that first fateful track meet.

"Well, in the masters competition, you compete in five-year age groups, so I can set a lot of records," he said modestly. "But if there was an open division, I wouldn't be anything. Now I've outlived most of my competition, so most anything I run is a new world record! Still, they're rapidly being wiped out by some really good runners coming up behind me."

For all of his victories, Paul said his first two marathons have given him his biggest thrills in running—so far. The first was in Goteberg, Sweden, in 1977; the second was a year later in Northern California.

"At the World Masters Championship in Goteborg, I'd run several distance races and was feeling pretty good, so I decided to try the marathon," he said. "I ran the marathon and overtook the champion five miles from the finish. Then I was afraid he would catch me and pass me—but he never did. That was the first marathon I'd ever run and I won it and became the new age-group champion. The time was four hours and four minutes.

"But I guess the next race gave me an even bigger thrill. It was the first and only time I broke four hours in the marathon. The time was 3:59, so I just barely broke it. It was on the Avenue of the Giants in Northern California.

"I guess those two races probably stand out more than anything else because that's quite an achievement for a kid who had never been able to do anything until he happened into masters running—I call it geriatric running."

Paul makes it sound easy, but the road to running fame and success has been anything but easy. Paul and his first wife divorced in the 1960s and he later married his college sweetheart. He was devastated when she died from Alzheimer's disease in 1982.

"Running has meant everything to me, especially after my wife died," he told *The New York Times*.

Also along the way he's had five cataract surgeries, and three lens implants.

"And I broke my wrist one morning running," he said. "I was doing some speed intervals on the track at 4 a.m. and I had just opened up to my best speed when someone left a hurdle down that I didn't see. I tripped over that and broke my right wrist when I fell.

"I have several doctors interested in my level of physical fitness and some of them check me from time to time. They are quite amazed at what I've accomplished. They are very supportive and wish there were more people taking care of their bodies like I am. They don't tell me what to do—I know what to do! But they check the results. They check my blood pressure, my weight, my cholesterol, my oxygen capacity, and all that sort of stuff."

Paul is equally serious about his diet.

"I'm not a strict vegetarian, but I tend to lean to the vegetarian side," he said. "I don't eat as much meat as I did before. I've tried to cut the fat from my diet, emphasize fruit, vegetables, legumes, and grains. I'm particular about getting plenty of fiber in my diet. Just the things anybody ought to do.

"Since I tend towards being vegetarian, I also do the things that are necessary when you are depending on vegetables for your proteins. You have to have your grains and your legumes at the same meal to get all of the amino acids you need to build protein. When you exercise as much as I do, you don't need to be so strict about your diet—you can cheat a little—well, maybe I cheat a lot—but still my cholesterol is low, and my weight is pretty steady."

Still, Paul admits that good health isn't the only reason he runs. There are other reasons, reasons relating to self-esteem, a sense of accomplishment, and—well—*pride.*

"It does something for my ego, it gives me a sense of accomplishment," he said. "I'm doing something that few people do and that gives me a sense of pride, so there's that angle."

That sense of accomplishment is another reason why he prefers masters competitions to open meets.

"It all should be by age group, even up to 110, if anybody is going to keep running until they're 110," Paul said. "I've been faced with that problem ever since I began running. I've been complaining when they have a meet and say, '60 and over.' I can't compete with 60-year-olds. Heck, I didn't start running until I was 67 and I'm still not fast—and I'm getting slower all the time now. If I had to compete with the 60- or 70-year age groups, I'd never have a chance to win and there would be no incentive for me to go to the expense of going to these meets!

"Winning does something for one's ego. If you don't have

the five-year age groups for all us old pugs, then we're not going to go to your meet. I've got an invitation for a meet in Palo Alto and the top bracket is 70-plus. I won't go to their meet. I might go as an invited guest, but I won't go to compete in it. I won't enter any meets anymore unless they have five-year age groups up to 100."

Paul is equally adamant that people in their 70s, 80s, 90s, and more, can do anything he is currently doing. Including running marathons.

He said that more than 12 percent of the entrants in the recent New York Marathon were over the age of 50. There were more than 400 who were 60 or older.

"There's no reason why they can't start to take care of themselves; they can always improve their condition," he said. "They may not reach the peak that they want, but they can always improve and feel better for it. Of course, the earlier they start, the more assured they'll be of success."

That's much the same advice he gives younger people.

"I say, 'Keep in shape, and keep on doing what you're doing,'" Paul said. "In other words, the earlier you start to adjust to a proper lifestyle, the more assured you will be of the rewards that are there for you.

"When I first started lecturing, I realized that most of the things you can do to prevent coronary heart disease apply to a lot of cancers as well—so I brought that in.

"Then I realized that the whole thing was a matter of a lifestyle. You can control a lot of catastrophies that tend to overtake people when they get to be my age. You minimize that. I think at least half of all cancer can be prevented and I'm sure 90 percent of all coronary heart disease is preventable. People aren't aware of that until I point out the evils of the things they're doing wrong.

"The things I bring up include improper diet, too much fat, a lack of regular exercise, the abuse of nicotine, alcohol, and caffeine, and a lack of fiber. That's the essence of my whole presentation."

Paul's presentations have such titles as "Life Styling for Health, Happiness and Zestful Longevity" and have the additional weight of authority in that—besides the fact there are not many 93-year-olds still able to run marathons—he is a medical doctor with expertise in nutrition and wellness.

"Other doctors pat me on the back when they realize that what I'm doing is the proper thing," he said. "Quite a few do it. You'll see fewer and fewer doctors smoking now. It's remarkable. You can go to a medical meeting and almost none of the doctors are smoking. And most have got their weight under control, too—although some of them are still big. But most of them are working on their weight control and diet because they know that the serious diseases that were thought to be diseases of old age are *not* diseases of old age at all—but diseases of improper lifestyle.

"I do a lot lecturing. I'm trying to tell the world how to live properly so they'll live forever."

Paul has a powerful incentive, if not to live forever, then to live to age 100 and beyond. He wants to run and complete the New York Marathon when he is 100.

"There is a $100,000 prize and nobody's done it yet," he told the *Los Angeles Times*. "I actually think I have a good chance of making 110.

"My only mission in life now," he told *The New York Times*, "is to convince people this is possible. With proper living, they can eliminate coronary heart disease. I can't see. I can't hear. And I have no teeth"—he was exaggerating more than a bit— "but if I couldn't run, I'd be under sod right now."

Chapter 21

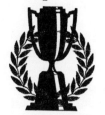

Hazel Stout

PORTLAND, OREGON—What's this perfectly nice little grandmother doing talking about bungee jumping? And worse, what's she doing actually *going* alpine sledding? Or white-water rafting? Or—heavens to Betsy!—sky diving?

For 89-year-old Hazel Stout, Portland's best-known senior thrill-seeker, it's all in a day's work.

Her various activities have earned her appearances on shows like "Late Night with David Letterman," "Gary Collins" and others, all of whom were smitten by her old-fashioned charm and wide-eyed innocence.

"Oh, Letterman was a lot a lot of fun," Hazel said. "Not so much happened on the show, but the staff before I went in were all so fabulous to me. He was real nice. I understand that he can be abrasive; he certainly wasn't with me. I enjoyed it because they treat you so nicely. They send a limo to take you where you need to go, they provide a lovely hotel room, they even paid for my daughter to go back with me.

"He showed a tape of my jump, and when I stepped to the doorway, he said, 'Who's that pushing you out of the plane? I think we should take that up with the DA.'"

Hazel smiled a somewhat confused, but still beatific, smile.

Earlier, a reporter from NBC had watched the jump and said, "What's the matter with your family? Are they trying to get rid of you? Have you got a lot of money?"

Hazel looked shocked at the thought.

"I said, 'Oh *no*! My family is *precious*, and they've always loved me dearly. I *know* they don't want to get rid of me.'"

Growing up in an active family, Hazel was expected to keep up with her brothers. When she was five, her 10-year-old brother took her by her bathing suit and tossed her into the water to sink or swim. That was her only swimming lesson.

"Except for the exercises I've always done, and the calisthenics I do at home, about the only regular exercise I've ever gotten has been swimming, which I always like to do, just for fun, a couple times a week," she said.

"My husband Waldo liked to swim, too. When he was alive, we used to go two or three times a week in the summertime. We'd go out to the Columbia River to Rooster Rock and we would swim there. I don't really like pools, I don't like the chlorine water, so I don't do much of that any more."

Walking hand in hand, Waldo and Hazel Stout were a familiar sight for many years at Portland's museums, art galleries, operas, and symphony concerts. Hazel still talks about him with a mixture of respect and longing.

"We were married for 48 years and we really had an idyllic life together—the romance never went out of it," she said. "It was just a very happy time. I attribute my good health and my outlook to the kind of life I had with him. He's been gone 15 years. Waldo died on the seventh day of the seventh month of 1977. So I've never considered seven a very lucky number.

"But he was fortunate in a way. He was 83 and had never been sick. I just couldn't imagine him ever being sick. But about 10 p.m. that night he put his hand across his stomach and said 'Oh.' That was all he said. By the time I got to him, he didn't even know me. He had an aneurysm. It burst. I've always been so grateful that he did live to be 83 and was never sick and didn't have to suffer the pains of old age."

Hazel, then 73, was grief-stricken and stayed at home for days.

"Before he died, I used to think, 'If anything happened to Waldo, I wouldn't be able to survive. I wouldn't have any interests,'" she said.

"Fortunately, about a month or so after Waldo died, a friend we had known a long time said, 'Hazel, it's time you learned another side of life. I'm going to teach you how to fish and how to do a lot of things.' And he did! He stepped in and was really kind of a life saver for me.

"He taught me how to fish, and we went to Hawaii, and we went up in a glider. We went to Hawaii three different times, which was great fun. Then when we went back to visit his folks in Michigan, he taught me how to ice fish and snowmobile, how to go down the slides in the New Hampshire mountains, and just do a lot of fun things I'd never done. So I really started all over again. A lot of my fun started when I was 73."

But to go from art shows and recitals to daydreaming about skydiving or white-water canoeing? Isn't that something of an abrupt change of pace?

"I never even gave it a thought before because Waldo was very protective of me," she said gaily. "He was 10 years older and he would have just died if I had told him I was going to jump out of an airplane! Every time I'd go out without him, which was very rarely because we were always together, he would say, 'Be careful crossing the street!'"

"If my husband was still alive, he'd think I was crazy," she told the Associated Press. "He'd have had me committed if I said I wanted to jump out of a plane."

Over the next 16 years, Hazel began to try the different sporting, athletic—even daredevil—activities that appealed to her.

"Riding in the glider in Hawaii didn't take any skill from me," she said. "They pull a plane up, then cut it loose, and you just glide with a pilot over the ocean, over the mountains. It was really fun. It was usually a two-person glider, but because the pilot was a she, we had three. It goes by weight, if I'd been any heavier, we couldn't have gone with three. But I weigh 100 pounds.

"I did go up in a hot air balloon in 1982 and I went alpine sledding in 1979–80. Coming down the slides, that's exciting— but it wasn't risky or dangerous. It's not like the Winter Olympics bobsledding, not at all. I haven't done anything *that* daring."

In May of 1992 she went white-water rafting, something she'd been looking forward to for years.

"I thought it would be real wild," she said. "But the water was low, so it wasn't as exciting as I had wanted it to be.

"Right now I'm considering bungee jumping—but my family doesn't want me to do it. They think it is too dangerous. Somebody told me that the jolt when you jump isn't any more than when a parachute opens. I had visions of maybe snapping my spine or something."

But the single event that garnered Hazel the most attention was skydiving on her 88th birthday. She says much of the credit belongs to a granddaughter who lives in Santa Fe, New Mexico, and her sky-diving husband Rick.

"I was in Santa Fe when my granddaughter said, 'Portland'— all my grandkids call me Portland—'why don't you do something exciting on your birthday?'

"I said, 'Like what?'

"She said, 'Sky dive with Rick.' Rick is an aeronautical

engineer who also teaches flying and sky dives as a hobby. He just loves it. I said I'd think about it.

"So I came home and as my birthday got nearer, I thought, 'That *would* be fun.'"

So Hazel celebrated her birthday at the drop zone at Mendota, California, and at 10,500 feet *above* Mendota.

"This was a tandem jump; you don't have to have training," she said. "You *do* have to sign an awful lot of papers and listen to a tape of the dangers you might encounter. But that was all. Then you get suited up and just do it!"

It took the little airplane 20 minutes to reach 10,500 feet above the drop zone.

"If it hadn't been for Rick, I guess I might have been more scared," Hazel said. "He kept patting me and talking to me the whole time we were going up. So I pretty well knew what it would be like when I stepped out. When you jump, I will say, it looks like a long way down, but I really wasn't too frightened. Maybe because I had so much confidence in him. And I know my granddaughter wouldn't let me do it if it were dangerous.

"As I fell, I was thinking how beautiful it was. We free fell for 40 seconds, which doesn't sound like much, but when you're falling—it is. Then we pulled the parachute and drifted on down for another five minutes. In free falling, I didn't have the sensation of falling at all, it is just like you are floating up there—even though you are falling at a rate of something like 120 miles an hour. But you don't have that sensation.

"My granddaughter told me, 'Now Portland, when you jump out, don't close your eyes—look around! Take in the whole scenery.' And I did."

Hazel hasn't done anything quite that intense since—much to her obvious disappointment.

"I thought the white-water rafting was going to be daring, but I guess you'd have to go down to Colorado to find some excitement there," she said. "And I went canoeing with the mayor of Portland once. So I guess those are about the only exciting things I've done lately. I've gotta think of something! Maybe bungee jumping—I'm really seriously contemplating that!"

In the meantime, while Hazel waits for her next hair-raising feat, she pays careful attention to her physical condition so she'll be ready.

"I've always tried to take care of myself and eat right," she said. "Another granddaughter, the one who lives here in Portland, is a dentist and she says, 'Now Portland, be sure and tell them that you are very careful about your diet, that you eat very healthful foods!' I can't really say that I've concentrated on that. I'm not a food fanatic, but I've never smoked. I will take a cocktail once in a while if I have company and they want one. It's not a habit, though. My husband and I both lived a healthful type of life.

"I'm not a vegetarian now, but I'm getting more that way the more I see what they do to meat. I just saw a program yesterday about beef that's imported. The inspection is practically nil. Let me tell you, it wasn't very appetizing. It would turn you off to meat. It seems like everyone you talk to is thinking about vegetarianism.

"I have never eaten many desserts—I just don't care too much for sugar. Well, I like a little tiny bit, a very moderate amount. Now, I've always liked butter and my granddaughter said, 'Don't tell you eat butter! That's bad!' She's so health conscious about food and she's not as healthy as I am! I think anything in moderation is OK."

Physically, Hazel says she's never felt better. She takes pills occasionally for high blood pressure and she continues to take daily vitamins.

"I've always taken a lot of vitamins, both my husband and I did," she said. "I don't know if that has anything to do with it, but I was 89 in August 1992, so it certainly hasn't hurt me any!

"My doctors, they're great. One wanted a tape of my jump, he was just so thrilled about the whole thing. I always know when I come in the office, he acts as if he's meeting a celebrity or something."

Hazel *is* something of a celebrity in Portland. In addition to her well-chronicled romantic punt with the mayor, she's appeared numerous times on local television and radio shows and in the local newspaper. She's also a much-in-demand speaker for school and civic groups. Young and old alike stop her on the street to ask advice or just to talk.

"That's a very rewarding thing when it does happen," Hazel said. "I have so many young people say, 'You're such an inspiration to me. If I could just be like you at your age.' Well, there's no reason why they can't be. It's just a matter of attitude. By thinking young, you're not going to turn the clock back, that's for sure. But if you think young and keep an interest in doing things, then you're going to stay young. Take Bob Hope: he and I are the same age. George Burns, of course, has got us beat, but he *does* things. How many *daring* things he does, I don't know—but he keeps active, anyway!"

She's also stopped by people nearing retirement age, people tired of sitting around watching TV or waiting for their children to call. They, too, want to be as active as she is at 89.

"As I said, I tell them it's all a matter of attitude," she said. "I've seen people who were old at 50 or 60, and some at 70 or 80—you have a choice. You can sit in a rocking chair waiting for time to go by and drop dead. Or you can take an interest in things.

"I know this sounds unbelievable because I'm 89, but I still love to shop for clothes. I love to go to the beauty shop and I just have an interest in living like other people who are not 89.

"So many people just lose interest. I say you have two choices, either lose interest or go the other way."

Hazel, obviously, has chosen that "other way." Her cheerful spirit is infectious, even to people who are meeting her for the first time. She says that much of the credit for her outlook goes to her family.

"I have, for instance, a wonderfully positive, optimistic daughter—I just have the one child—and I've never seen that girl with an unhappy look," Hazel said. "I said to her one time, 'How can you always look so cheerful and so happy?'

"She said, 'Well, mother, I guess I have so much to be happy about.' She's happily married, and they'll celebrate their 50th wedding anniversary in 1993.

"My good fortune is due so much to my family. It is a wonderful family and I just knew all my life that I was loved. That means so much. And I was fortunate to inherit good genes. I think what you're given you're supposed to take care of to the best of your ability."

In the end, Hazel says people of all ages can only be happy by living, *really living*, every minute to its fullest.

"Of course, there's a lot of things I'd still like to do, but I know better," she said. "I know I can't go windsurfing on the Hood River, for instance. "It's the windsurfing capital of the world, but I know that I can't because it takes a lot of upper-body strength. My granddaughter says it does, anyway. She said, 'Portland, you can't do that, you're not strong enough.' But I would still love to do it.

"I'd like to water-ski. It might be something to do, too. And I've thought about scuba diving, too. Now *that* might be fun.

"Just go ahead and do it. If there's something you want to do, just go ahead and do it! I'm saying that—and now I'm thinking about that bungee jumping again!"

Uh oh. Maybe it's time to call Letterman again

Chapter 22

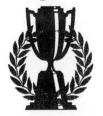

"Ginny" Wagner

SUN LAKES, ARIZONA—Maybe you've seen the Dancin' Grannies on "Donahue," or "This Morning with Gary Collins," or "Sally Jessy Raphael," or even "Arsenio." Maybe you remember them from the telecasts of the Fiesta Bowl Parade or Macy's Thanksgiving Day Parade. Or perhaps you've seen one of their three aerobic videos or the article in *USA Today*.

But if you've seen them, you know the truth in what founder Beverly Gemigniani says: "My choreography is still designed to get wolf whistles."

It's hardly an enlightened feminist attitude in 1992, but these Grannies don't seem to mind.

Many of those wolf whistles are directed at 72-year-old Virginia "Ginnie" Wagner. And in response, she kicks a little higher and smiles a little brighter. Clearly, Ginnie Wagner is having a ball.

"I was born in Iowa, moved to Wisconsin, and then to Michigan," she said. "I was married, but lost my husband to an automobile accident and was widowed at the age of 32. Then I was single for five years. I remarried after that. But I lost him to a heart attack. I've been a widow for the past 17 years—and I think I am going to stay that way."

Her second husband owned a restaurant near Detroit and the two ran it together, walking the dining area, overseeing the kitchen, running the cash register. It was a lot of hard work.

"Then, when I had had enough of that at the age of 60, I decided to retire," she said. "I had four children who were all on their own and I said, 'Now it's time for me.' I liked Michigan, but I didn't like the weather—very humid in the summer and very cold and snowy in the winter. I decided I wanted to change that and move somewhere with a steadier climate."

In 1982, Ginnie chose Phoenix, Arizona, partly because of the weather, and partly because she had—and still has—a daughter who lives in the Phoenix area.

"But at age 60, I was not in such good shape," she said. "I had smoked for 30 years, but I gave up smoking in 1975 because I was feeling the effects. I realized that I was not in such great shape. I'd walk a while and get very much out of breath. I was heavier, too. So that's when I decided I'd better do something.

"I took an inventory and decided I want to grow old gracefully. I don't want to be dumpy and dowdy. Then I decided, right then and there: exercise."

Even though she had worked hard in her restaurant and was on her feet all day, it wasn't an aerobic workout. So the first thing she did in Phoenix was look for a workout program.

She found a new program started by another recent arrival to Phoenix, Beverly Gemigniani.

"I found that it took me a period of a year before I could get myself into the position of being able to do some of these steps without practically dying out there," Ginnie said. "The next thing that came was to lose weight, because I was much heavier then. I found that by carrying this extra weight around I wasn't helping myself, I couldn't do these things. So I went into Weight Watchers."

Ginnie said that the more Beverly taught aerobics, the more she knew she needed to study fitness. Beverly's first step was to complete the study necessary for International Dance Exercise Association certification.

"That's when this thing kind of evolved," Ginnie said. "Since we are in a big retirement area, we had between 10 and 20 people when Beverly initially started. We have a lot of groups around here and after a while they'd say, 'Won't you come and show us what you do?' So that's how we got started, by gosh and by golly!"

By gosh and by golly, indeed! Within months, the Dancin' Grannies found themselves invited to perform throughout Arizona. They also discovered that a *lot* of ladies wherever they went wanted to be Grannies.

"You have to be at least 60 or older, you have to be a grandmother, and you have to be a member here at Sun Lakes Retirement Community," Ginnie said. "There haven't been any auditions because we are primarily the original group that started. We have taken on two other girls in the past year or two. They were members of the exercise class and so I guess by way of that Beverly was able to see how fit they were, so that they would be able to continue in our program."

Word of the Dancin' Grannies soon spread outside of Arizona. They competed in the Senior Olympics and Ginnie won a gold medal in her age group for solo performance.

"It was a tremendous challenge for me just getting up there all by myself," she said. "You're being judged on how well you use your body, what forms of exercises you're doing, and how well you're doing them. Fortunately, Bev is a very talented person in her own right and she does all of the choreography for the group."

Next came invitations to participate in several well-known holiday parades.

"This was not just walking down the street," Ginnie said. "We were aerobicizing. The least amount we would do was two miles, and eventually we went up to four. We have paraded in different cities in Arizona, then we did the Fiesta Bowl, and then we were invited to do Macy's Thanksgiving Day Parade. That was a tremendously exciting experience; you have to be in extremely good shape to do this.

"There are just 10 of us in the Dancin' Grannies, but when we do the parades, we bring in 15 other gals to train, and call them the Parade Grannies."

From the parades came appearances on the various television programs. Ginnie's favorite TV appearance, perhaps because it was her first, was "Donahue."

"I guess because this was a person I had seen on TV," she said. "This was a celebrity! I was just so thrilled knowing and realizing that when I got up on that screen, I was going to be viewed by millions of people. It was a little scary.

"But I will say that Donahue really put us at ease; he was a very nice fellow. We got through it and got through it beautifully. Yeah, that was exciting. And as they came along after that, then we knew what to expect. But that was our very first experience with any kind of studio."

Armed with the positive response from the network shows, Beverly decided the time was right to tape an exercise video with the Grannies.

"We wanted the older people out there to see the importance of doing exercise—even if it is even the most simple exercise," Ginnie said. "Beverly wanted to show them that you can do it right. So we have now done four videos. The fourth was taped in September 1992."

But Ginnie says that, more than the new-found fame and attention, she's treasured the personal growth that's accompanied the Dancin' Grannies' success.

"I think all the way along it has been a growing experience for me," she said. "This exercise and being involved has opened doors and broadened my life to where my attitude turned away from age as an ominous part of my path of life to a different way of thinking, to feeling younger and growing older gracefully. I've increased my endurance and toned up my body and gone to Weight Watchers and lost 20 pounds—which enables me to move more freely.

"I did not want to be just a lovable, plump, little grey-haired lady whose life consists of pushing a vacuum cleaner and hauling a basket of laundry all day, a workhorse whose figure—even with that heavy lifting—has gotten away from her. I was able to firm myself up. I feel younger and my outlook has improved.

"I don't think of my age. I'm in my 72nd year, but that doesn't mean anything to me."

With that increased personal awareness has come a new surge of confidence. The once-shy Ginnie has begun traveling the country and performing and lecturing at Senior Expos.

"At the Expositions, we have to be our own emcees," she said. "We do a three-minute dance—and it is one that will take your breath away—and then afterwards we talk about ourselves. It's gotten me over a lot of stage fright. I was always a little shy, now I can take the challenge and push out there—which is good. It makes you feel young again.

"You are up in front of people, you are talking to your own peer group and you are demonstrating to your own peer group. It so amazing. You get such an elated feeling when they come up to you after you've done this and say, 'Oh look: I'm doing this... and I walk, and I exercise.'

"So you realize that now we have created somewhat of a role model and we have a mission. That mission is to tell those people, even though they may have some physical impairment that keeps them back, at least they're trying and at least they're not going to the rocking chair."

Watching Ginnie's energetic performance on the Dancin' Grannies videos, it's hard to imagine that she even *owns* a rocking chair! Still, she says exercise alone didn't give her a star-quality figure at age 72.

"I watch my fat intake, I watch the quantity of food I eat, and I eat more fruits and vegetables. I also stick with the chicken and fish," she said. "Well, I had always been a meat eater and I've tried to cut that out of my diet, but occasionally I'll have a little red meat. But mainly I've learned to watch the amount that I eat. If I feel like I'd like to have a little meat, I will. But I don't have it as often as I used to."

As important as diet, as important even as exercise, Ginnie believes, is attitude. *Doing* all the right things isn't necessarily enough. The change has to be deeper still.

"Before I began getting in shape, I was primarily being put in the position of raising my family by myself," she said. "I was too consumed with my family and it just took away from myself. Now that I have that responsibility lifted from me, and I've taken stock of my own self—it's been so much better for me because I can go ahead and feel free to do what I want to.

"It takes a little doing. You can get a little lazy when you get this age. You can take a look at yourself and say, 'It's time for you to take it easy—you've worked hard all your life.' But it doesn't really help you in the long run because you only become more depressed when you realize that, in your December years, your shelf life isn't all that long. We have to keep going and work to have the quality of life we want."

Ginnie says there is yet another component of a changed life. It involves a spiritual change as well. For the Grannies themselves. For their audience.

"Before we give any performance at all, we say a prayer," she said, "because we feel that we have a motive. I guess this is where the faith part comes in—that we must give to someone else the gift that has been given to us. We always encircle ourselves before we start a performance and we ask God to help us motivate those people and help us to show them the right way. I guess it has been inspirational in that regard.

"You have to stick together; we're almost like sisters now. We do a lot of practicing. When we are getting ready for a video, we work six days a week. So you get to see these gals. A lot.

"It's been a stimulus in my life. Otherwise, I think I would just kind of die on the vine. I'm not the kind of person who can sit still. You can go out and play cards with the girls just so long—or even play golf. It's been just a wonderful, wonderful camaraderie with the gals. It has been the stimulus that's kept me going. I think if I ever had to leave, I'd have quite an adjustment."

Perhaps that's one of the secrets of the Dancin' Grannies' popularity. They adjust attitudes. But even a great idea won't succeed if the marketplace isn't convinced that the inventor doesn't truly believe in his or her idea.

The Grannies believe. Every one of them. And that belief comes through, whether they are performing in person or aerobicizing on "Arsenio."

"When I reached 50, I thought it was the end of the world," Ginnie said. "And I told my husband at the time, 'This is going to be a tremendous milestone. I just don't want to hit that 50 mark.' But as I passed it and when I got to 70, 70 didn't faze me at all.

"Now people recognize us from the videos, which is really quite an astounding thing. Because we don't look at ourselves in that way. We're just plain, ordinary women. I guess if you have travelled and if you have been on TV, someone must see you because they're always saying, 'Oh, I saw you on "Donahue!"' It's a good feeling to know that at least we've been out there and people are recognizing us and saying, 'I've heard of the Grannies. Yes, I've seen you!' That's a really good feeling."

Naturally, with that increased exposure has come increased responsibility. Both by accident and by choice, Ginnie and the other Grannies have found themselves cast as experts in the field of senior fitness.

"I wouldn't call myself an expert. However, I do keep myself abreast of all the different things," Ginnie said. "Whenever there is an article, I read it and try to keep myself up on all these things so that I'm doing the right thing. I guess maybe you could call me some kind of a specialist, since I've been coached in the proper use of my body. And hopefully I can pass some of this knowledge on to other people."

So what is her response when a younger person comes up and asks, "Ginnie, what do I need to do to be as active as you are at 72?"

"I would tell that younger person to watch their diet, to work out, and to exercise," she said. "A lot of them do a lot of sitting in front of the TV. Get them involved in sports and, as they grow up, they will become so in tune with the need for an energetic life, they won't drop out."

And her advice for a person nearing retirement age who

wants to regain—or discover for the first time—an active, vital lifestyle in their 60s, 70s, and beyond?

"I'd tell them just about the same thing," Ginnie said. "First of all, look at yourself and find out, 'What do I need to get myself going?' A lot of them don't feel that they would continue with an exercise program. So, at that point, I would say, 'What you need is to get a buddy system and the two of you do it together. And don't expect miracles overnight, it's going to take a while. If you monitor each other, you will keep going. And once you see that you are progressing with it, nothing will stop you.'

"So they need to get, first of all, that feeling of motivation. And that's where we feel we come in. When they see that we can do this, when they see we've kept our weight down, they generally say, 'If you can do it, I can do it too.'

"I just tell them to go ahead and keep working and not to look at themselves as being older."

There are, of course, some physical ailments that no amount of exercise can overcome. Ginnie admits that she's been fortunate. Her health has always been excellent.

"But we do have Grannies who have had quite extensive health problems," she said. "We have one gal who has rheumatoid arthritis, and her doctor explained to her that unless she kept her body going, she'd end up in a wheelchair. We have another gal who had open heart surgery and after she came home from the hospital, she came to class two weeks later and started doing exercises in her chair! We've got yet another gal who has back problems.

"I've been very lucky in regard to my health. The only serious health problem I've ever had was when I was 6 years old. Since then, I've always bounced back; I'm a very strong person. But I've been very lucky, too."

Perhaps. But for the oldest Dancin' Granny, luck is only one small facet of the total package. Confidence. Exercise. Diet. Attitude. A willingness to change. Faith. Luck.

"I'm caring for my 96-year-old mother," Ginnie Wagner said. "If heredity has anything to do with it, I hope to keep going for a number of years yet. She's still doing very well now, so maybe I have a few good genes."

The genes *must* be pretty good. Just ask the guys with the wolf whistles on Fifth Avenue each Thanksgiving.

Chapter 23

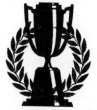

James R. Ward

SEMINOLE, FLORIDA—It was a cold, raw, drizzly September day in 1988, when James R. Ward attempted his first Tri-Fed/ USA Olympic distance triathlon in Wilkes-Barre, Pennsylvania. At age 71, he entered the 70-and-over age bracket.

"That morning it was cold and rainy," Jim recalled. "During the heat of the day, it only got up to 57. When we started that morning with the swim, it was only in the high 40s and a cold rain continued all day long on the course through the mountains. It just washed out everything.

"When I finished the run, I was still blue. All of my opponents had by then dropped out, fearing hypothermia, although I didn't know that at the time.

"When I finished, instead of waiting to see how I placed, I went to my car, drove half an hour back to my hotel in Wilkes-Barre. And when I ran by the front desk, I called out, 'Have somebody send up a pot of hot coffee as soon as possible!' When I got to my room, I filled up the tub with hot water and soaked it up and drank hot coffee until I thawed out.

"Then I dressed in dry clothes and drove all the way back to the site of the meet where they were just reading out the results.

"That's when I discovered I'd won my first national championship."

Jim received the news with the same stoic air of casual aplomb that has marked all of the events of his life. After all, it takes something pretty significant to excite someone who has been a war hero in two wars, featured in his own Armor All commercial, a published author, and a marathon champion.

And the Tri-Fed/USA Championship? It was only the first of seven through early 1992 for the seemingly indestructible Mr. Ward.

Born in Bayonne, New Jersey, on August 31, 1917, Jim grew up in Malden, Massachusetts. He wasn't a particularly athletic kid, or so he recalls.

"I used to hang around with a couple of guys and we'd play 'follow the leader,'" he said. "We were constantly daring one another to do things like standing on your hands atop the flagpole in front of the First Baptist Church! Or hanging by our knees from another flagpole that was in front of a department store in Malden, Massachusetts, five stories above the ground. Then we began hanging by our heels! Eventually they took that flagpole down. The police used to chase us up on the roof. It was just mischief, but it was a lot of fun when you're 12–13 years old. We also learned how to walk on our hands quite well."

Jim attended Boston College and eventually received a degree in economics. At various times during high school and college, he worked as a farmhand, lumberjack, bus driver, lecturer on sightseeing buses, and even as an oil refinery worker.

When World War II broke out, Jim entered the U.S. Army as a private. But, because of his proficiency in foreign languages, he was quickly recruited from the parachute infantry by the OSS. In time, he found himself near Alegyun, Burma, 10–12 miles due west of Pinwe in northern Burma.

It was the beginning of a harrowing 13-month stint behind Japanese Army lines as commander of a native guerrilla force.

Jim said his Burmese tribesmen were brilliant jungle fighters. They needed to be. One of their major campaigns was to relieve the British 36th Division, which was being detained by two regiments of the Japanese 18th division in a network of heavily reinforced concrete bunkers. Jim's orders were to meet with a battalion of the Chinese National Army and take some of the heat off the British.

"I was told that, at a certain place about halfway between where the British were and where we were, the Chinese would show up at a certain village and meet me," Jim said. "We'd establish contact and work out our signals. I spoke a little Chinese—very little—and I took a patrol and went over there.

"And as we were in the outskirts of the village, one of my tribesmen, who was crawling through the jungle just to my side, starting saying 'Japanese, Japanese.'

"I said, 'No, it has to be Chinese. The Chinese are supposed to meet us here.' I couldn't see anything that seemed all that suspicious to me, although those tribesmen can tell when a leaf is turned the wrong way on a tree in the jungle. And in what looked to me like jungle and bushes, he could see a camouflaged position. So I figured it was Chinese.

"So I stood up in the road and said in Chinese, 'I am an American soldier'. Just about that time, I saw the bushes about 150 yards in front of me starting to move and then a host of rifles pointing at me. I still thought it was Chinese until a barrage of shots rang out and my guerrillas started opening up in return fire and I was caught in the middle!

"So I took a flying leap—and my troops later said it was the biggest jump they had ever seen anyone take in all of their lives—I leapt 20 feet into the rice-paddy fields, rolled over, and crawled back through the rice to where my men were."

Shaken, Jim survived. He also figured in a nasty firefight in October 1944 when the Japanese tried to overrun his base camp near Alegjun.

"About 3 a.m., the Japanese came in using cold steel—bayonets and swords—rather than firing at us," Jim said. "We figure they were trying to save their ammunition because they wanted to go around us and try to hit the rear of the 36th.

"They probed and broke through our lines in a couple of places. For about 30 minutes there was a helluva battle there and everything kept growing more and more confusing. So finally I had to give the order to pull out. I tried to lead a counterattack back in, but I got caught in the middle.

"We finally got out. It was a very bad situation, and it was the worst defeat any of our outfits had, but we stopped the Japanese probe."

Jim ended the war as a captain and continued as a reserve officer, eventually reaching the rank of lieutenant colonel. He then worked for the U.S. Foreign Service, with overseas service as a consular or reporting officer in embassies or consulates in Kuala Lampur (1948–50), Rangoon (1950–53), Tokyo (1954–56), Vienna (1960–62), Prague (1962–65), Vietnam (1966–68), Vientiane (1970–72), and Port of Spain (1972–74).

In Vietnam, Jim was in charge of most of the pacification apparatus in the Delta region of that war–torn country.

"The war there was the struggle for the political control of the population," Jim said. "The Viet Cong were trying to get control through persuasion or, if that didn't work, through intimidation. Our job was to try to win the population over to the side of the South Vietnamese. So it was a political effort much more than it was a military effort."

For his efforts—and eventually the Delta became one of the most secure areas in Vietnam—Jim received numerous citations and commendations. But he left something behind in Vietnam as well: The Wards' only son, First Lieutenant James Patrick Ward, was killed in action during the war.

Jim retired from the Foreign Service in the late 1970s, sold real estate in Maryland for a while, and eventually retired in 1980.

"My wife and I bought a motor home and toured from Vermont to Florida," he said. "We spent two months in Florida and criss-crossed the state. We settled in Seminole. We went to visit and stayed."

At first, Jim played a lot of golf and read of of lot books. He wrote a critique of what he believed had happened in Vietnam. He wrote a number of war-related articles. He even tried a novel about Vietnam, but it was obvious that he was not meant for a leisurely retirement.

"I love the game of golf, but it is more a game like bridge is a game," Jim said. "It isn't much exercise—particularly if you use carts. I discovered that while I could hit the ball a long way, and I got my average into the upper 70s, I didn't have the temperament for golf. I would get angry with myself. And in golf, the harder you try, the worse you do. You have to be able to concentrate and relax at the same time. I guess I was having difficulty doing that. I'd be shooting par through the 15th hole and then I'd blow up."

When all else failed, Jim would go jogging. As a reserve officer, he sometimes had to go on duty with various Special Forces units.

"If I wasn't in shape, they'd kill me," he said. "I discovered that the hard way. So I stayed in shape and kept running 10–12 miles a week. I stopped smoking in 1975, right after I retired from the government. After I stopped smoking, I started running more. I smoked mostly a pipe and cigars in those days and every time I wanted to smoke, I'd go out and run a hundred yards or so and the urge would disappear. So I increased my running about that time.

"I kept at that until I read in the paper about a group of older guys over 60 who were competitive in running. So I decided I'd try just to enter a race. So I entered that 10K race and I discovered that there were five of us over the age of 60. I came in fifth of the five. I talked to them and discovered that these guys were running between 40 and 60 miles a week. Here I was running about 12."

Nevertheless, Jim found that he liked not just the competition, but the training regimen required to run the longer races. In time, it became something close to a happy obsession with him.

"When I was 65, I ran my first marathon," Jim said. "I did a few more, maybe half a dozen at that time.

"Then, when I was turning 68, my wife asked me what I'd like for my birthday. I said a bicycle so I could try a triathlon, which was fairly new back then. I'd been hearing a lot about it, everybody was doing it, including some friends of mine who said they loved it—but they were all younger people.

"So in 1986 I did my first triathlon at age 68 after about six months of learning how to handle a bike. I liked it and I felt less tired after a triathlon than after a run for a comparable period of time because of the variety of exercise you get. So I started doing longer triathlons."

The next logical question is, of course, why the triathlon? There are a host of arduous sports and activities. Why the most grueling, exhausting, *macho* sporting event in the world?

"The cross-training is much better than just running," he said. "I was basically just a runner in the beginning. When I was training for marathons, my wife and daughter complained I was getting emaciated in my upper body. My average weight was 184 and I wasn't considered overweight at all. Then I got down to 160 when I was training full-time for marathons. So I decided to do some weight-lifting and that's when people began suggesting triathlons, where swimming works your upper body. I started swimming more and more and it did just that."

By the time he'd turned 70, Jim had pretty well established himself as the Florida champion in the over-65 age group—if not the over-60 crowd. It was that year—1988—that he entered, and won, the Tri-Fed/USA Triathlon in Wilkes-Barre.

"The next one that was memorable was the U.S.T.S. Olympic distance triathlon championships, sponsored by Bud Lite," Jim said. "They host about 12 triathlons per year, then have a final one. The championships were at Hilton Head Island, South Carolina. It was also memorable because of the cold and the strong winds—which hit about 20 knots."

In fact, the seas were so rough that the official swimming course had to be changed. The change also necessitated an additional two-mile walk for the competitors.

"Once we got up there, the waves were so bad and the current was so strong that it swept some of the pros inland!"

Jim said. "The waves were about five feet high. We got out about 250 yards, swimming straight out into the water so we could go far enough out to pass the buoy, when they sent a boat out after us and the mate said, 'You've already passed the buoy!'

"We had to swim a breaststroke to get on top of the waves so you could see the shore. I could see where the finish line was because it was near the hotel where I was staying. So I would aim for that. I'd swim hard for about 100 yards, stop and get on top of a wave again and see where the hotel was, and continue that way. With that fast current, I made the whole distance in 19 minutes. My God, that was the fastest swim I ever had!"

As Jim emerged from the water, his wife threw him a jacket to cover his nearly blue skin. He hopped on his bike and rode on, once again, to victory.

The classic Ironman Triathlon—a 2.4-mile swim, 112-mile bicycle ride, and a full 26.2-mile marathon—may be the toughest athletic event in the world. And Jim Ward has run nearly 50 triathlons in the past five years, winning virtually all of them.

It is something, he says, that requires preparedness on a military scale.

"To compete in the Ironman, you have to train a lot," he said. "In fact, I've been training sometimes as much as 24 hours a week—just running, swimming, and biking—but with some weight-lifting too, because you have to be in super all-around shape. I swim around 6,000–9,000 meters per week, run anywhere from 25 to 40 miles per week, and bike about 100 to 180 miles per week.

"Now I wouldn't do the same regimen every week. Some weeks I'd put more stress on the biking and less on the running, for example. But I try to get in the maximum swim every week."

Jim's family and his doctor have supported him in such a time commitment to the triathlons.

"My family doctor is a runner, though he doesn't compete," Jim said. "He used to be very heavy and now he's very slender and in good shape. He says it is rather amazing, the condition I'm in, especially my heart and lungs and my organs are in great shape and he encourages me to compete.

"Generally, my wife is quite happy, although at times she gets a little irked when she says she wants to do something and I say, 'Golly, I've got to get in my biking today!' But I try to accommodate her as much as possible. You have to hit a balance there. Frequently I yield on the training."

The more triathlons he's run, the more radically he's changed his diet as well. Jim said he's read constantly on the subject of nutrition.

"I find that I eat an awful lot more carbohydrates like grains, pasta, rice," he said. "I do eat meat, but nowhere near as much as I used to. If we have steak more than twice a month now, that's exceptional. I don't eat lightly, I eat a lot. And I drink an awful lot of water."

As Jim's exploits become more widely known through interviews and his recent Armor All commercial, he says he's suddenly found himself thrust into the position of spokesman for senior fitness. It's a position he's learned to relish.

"I get young people coming up to me a lot saying, 'Gee, my father can't do anything any more at your age. He's crippled with arthritis. How do you do it?'

"I say, 'Well, it's partly that I'm lucky, it's partly due to my genes, and it's also partly due to the fact that I've always been active,'" Jim said. "The expenditure of energy increases your energy levels.

"Another factor is that you need to be mentally interested. With my background, I'm very much interested in what's happening in the world. Sometimes my wife gets bored watching the news. But to me, it is a great big soap opera. I read a great deal, too."

Today, Jim Ward is often called to speak on fitness and health by groups of retired people in Florida. Again, it is a subject that he feels passionately about.

"I usually encourage them to start very, very gradually," he said. "Most people get real enthusiastic the first day when their energy levels are high. They run too fast, they run on their toes too much, then they get shin splints! But they feel real good that first day—and overdo it. I have to hold them back if I'm with them. I just encourage them to do things very gradually, to build up to a 20-minute walk—or a 20-minute walk every other day, depending on their age and condition.

"For somebody who is not really in good shape, I don't encourage anything more than a 20-minute walk every other day. When they show that they can handle that after a week or two, then maybe they can start doing it every day. Then do 30 minutes every other day. Then maybe jog 100 yards after a few weeks.

"The main thing is to build up very, very gradually. The worst thing you can do is overdo it at the beginning because that discourages people and they quit."

Not that "quit" is in Jim Ward's vocabulary. He is a confident, optimistic person, a tenacious competitor, a tireless health and fitness evangelist.

At the 1991 Tri-Fed/USA sprint distance triathlon in Aventura, Florida, a doctor was soliciting opinions from the competitors on the meaning of life. Jim was initially taken somewhat aback by the request, but quickly warmed to the challenge.

"When I got back, I sat down and wrote out some of the things I think about when I'm running," he said. "I do a lot of writing in my mind when I run, thinking about things I want to speak or write about. Philosophy is a subject I enjoyed in college.

"So I wrote a one-page paper and sent it to the doctor. He was very enthusiastic about the paper and sent a copy to the publisher of *Triathlon Today* and several other magazines.

"Essentially, I think the purpose of life is to live yourself and to propagate life. By living, I mean living life fully—not just existing—in every respect: mentally, physically, emotionally, and culturally. By propagating, I don't mean just begetting children, but also helping others to live their lives more fully."

Jim once carried a small tape recorder to record his thoughts while he ran, but the noise of the road—and his own breathing—made the tapes virtually unusable.

"So all I do now is jot down a few words to help me remember my thoughts when I sit down to transcribe them," he said. "Basically, I try to remember what I think about. I've found that after the second, sometimes the third, mile of running, I hit what's called the runner's high. You've run past that hill and can maintain a good speed and you're able to run real well and you feel you can run on indefinitely. And at that time, your mind is clearer and there's a period there when your mind works better than at any other time."

It's at that point that Jim tries to capture the abstract thoughts and feelings he's having as he runs, seemingly effortlessly, along yet another Florida back road.

In the end, he says his whole life is dedicated to striving for excellence, whether behind enemy lines in Burma, behind a desk in Prague, or behind a 30-year-old runner at the World Triathlon Championship in Avignon, France.

"That's sort of been ingrained in me," he said. "If I try to play golf, I try to be the best golfer I can be. I don't try to win just to beat other people. I am competitive by nature, but I just try to do the best I can do.

"After I'd been a triathlete after a couple of years, I decided to try to become the best I can be at my age because I enjoyed it. I also enjoy the traveling around.

"And, I just enjoy the competition. I guess I've always been goal-oriented. I tend to set goals for myself and have done so almost all my life. This is one more."

That, of course, all sounds very noble, very heroic, very stoic. But competing in the triathlons and marathons also gives Jim Ward one last competitive edge.

"When I go out and play some golf with old friends, when we're on the 15th hole and this guy says, 'Geez, my ass is dragging. I'm so tired. I'll be glad when this game is over,' I don't *dare* tell him that I swam a mile and a half and ran nine miles already that morning!"

Particularly not when there's two bits at stake on each hole!

Chapter 24

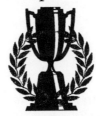

Dr. Fred White

DALLAS, TEXAS—At age 79, Dr. Fred White still gets *excited* about running. He's *passionate* about running. He once got so fired up on a trip to the Orient that he got on TV and offered a "flat-footed challenge" to the entire People's Republic of China, all two billion of 'em, to a foot race!

"There weren't any takers," he says somewhat apologetically, "although I don't think too many people watch TV over there."

Don't believe Fred couldn't have beat a few of them, too. To date, he's won 250 gold medals in state, regional, national, and international competition in a variety of sprints and field events. He's held a host of world records in the 70–74 and 75–79 age brackets, most recently the 60-yard-dash and the triple jump.

He also continues to teach at Dallas Baptist College, occasionally preaching on weekends, working on the Texas Senior Games board, and serving in a fund-raising and advisory capacity for various muscular dystrophy boards.

The lean, white-haired preacher comes from a family of athletes. One of 10 children—nine boys—of a Texas farmer, Fred was unbeaten in three years of running the mile at tiny Teneha High School. He also ran track at Baylor University in Waco, Texas.

"I've always stayed in good physical condition," Fred said. "I ran daily. I stayed with team sports through Baylor University and seminary, mostly in church leagues. About the only time I ever really got out of shape was when I was working on my doctorate and pastoring a church full time. That was about 1954, but I got back in good shape again.

"About 18 years ago, when I was 61 years old, I started taking this competitive running very seriously. I was still in really good shape then, but there was only one problem: I had to convert from a distance runner to a sprinter. It takes a totally different training program. As I gained speed, I lost the tremendous stamina I'd built up. You see, at age 60 I could run a six-minute mile.

"I switched to the sprints from the distances for two reasons: At 60, as busy as I was, I didn't have time to train for the distance events. It just takes an awful lot of running—eight to 10 miles a day—to get to a championship level. I didn't have time for that. The other thing was that I always knew that I could be a sprinter. With the time I had to put in on it and the fact that I was interested in the sprints, that's what determined it. I decided I'd go to it and it took two–three years before I could win on a national level."

His biggest hurdle to running sprints at age 60 wasn't the physical demands of the sport, but telling his wife Mary Lou what he was going to go.

"She always thought I was kind of an idiot anyway," Fred said cheerfully.

But even Mary Lou can't argue with Fred's success in track.

"I've done real well in recent years," he said. "I've won about everything I've entered. I haven't been beaten indoors at 55 meters in a long time. At a recent meet in Lubbock I ran the 55-meter, the 200-meter, and the 400-meter dashes. Last Saturday at an outdoor meet in Dallas I ran the 50-, 100-, 200- *and* 400-meter dashes. At the upcoming Dallas Senior Games, which is a full-scale track meet, I might do them all *and* the triple jump. It varies, depending on which events are which mornings.

"I'm in my last year in my age bracket of 75–79—I'm currently 79. Right now I'm losing to people like Payton Jordan, the former head track coach at Stanford, and Bill Winot, who just turned 75. I can't outrun either of them on an ordinary day right now. But next year I'll have just turned 80 and I'll be in a brand new age bracket and won't have them in my age bracket anymore. I ought to *really* clean up then."

There have been, of course, literally hundreds of meets in the past 20 years. A few have ended badly. During the 400-meter dash in the 1988 National Senior Championships, for instance, Fred tore a ligament in his right knee. And just after the Senior Olympics in Wisconsin, he had an eye operation to get a cataract removed and an implant put in.

But for the most part, Fred's running career has been an unbroken string of successes. Still, three meets come to mind:

"One took place in Atlanta, Georgia, about 12–13 years ago," he said. "I ran in the 200 meters, and outran a fellow from California and also a man from South Africa who was just a great competitor. Turns out, both of them were the world champions at the time and I outran them both and won that 200-meter dash!

"Then in San Juan, Puerto Rico, I won the 400-meter dash against an Australian runner who like to have killed me. It was the national championships and I had beaten the Australian fellow earlier at a meet at Rice University, so I was a little over-confident. When the race began, I was in lane six, and by the second curve he was way ahead of me, I just made up my mind, 'Either I'm going to win this race or die.'

"Of course, everybody in Puerto Rico cheers everybody *but* Americans, so the stands went wild when he raced ahead. Frankly, I didn't think I could catch him. But I got him the last two steps and the place went dead quiet. I also won the bronze in the triple jump at San Juan."

But Fred's fondest memory is from the 1985 World Masters Meet in Rome. Fred was part of a contingent of 35 Dallas senior athletes who—along with their wives and families—were inseparable during their stay in Italy.

"We all went over on the same flight, stayed in the same hotel, and got the same shaft once we got over there," he said. "I was, at that time, world champion in the 400-meter dash in my age bracket. But when I never made it beyond the first trial heat, I knew something was rotten in the state of Denmark and it was *all* rotten in Rome."

Despite a second-place finish in his heat, Fred's spot in the finals was awarded to an Italian runner. No amount of arguing could sway the Italian race officials. But Fred got a second chance to shine on the American relay team. The relays didn't have time trials or heats.

"We literally blew the rest of the world out on the relay," he said. "We won by 30 yards. It was really gratifying, especially since we had a new world record."

"I really enjoyed just being there, seeing the 60, 15-foot high white marble statues all around the periphery of the stadium. They were all perfect replicas of athletes in the nude and our wives kept asking us, 'Is *that* what a *real* athlete looks like?'"

Along the way, Fred's accomplishments have attracted the attention of both the media and some well-known physicians.

"I've been Dr. Kenneth Cooper's official guinea pig for the past 15 years," Fred said. "I come every year and go through his clinic. He doesn't charge me and I haven't missed a year yet. He does a detailed blood analysis, checks my triglycerides and cholesterol and such. He found the cholesterol was high, so my wife and I have gone on a low-fat diet. We're not slaves to what we eat, but we did get rid of the vast majority of the fats and sweets. Now we eat a well-balanced diet and my cholesterol is back to healthier levels, with the proper ratios of HDLs and LDLs.

"Other than having glaucoma in my left eye—for which I take one drop of medicine a day—Dr. Cooper has me on one vitamin a day. That's all the medicine I take.

"Dr. Cooper is really the only doctor I've ever had. When I've needed a shot or something, I've used my wife's doctor. I haven't been sick. Dr. Cooper is supportive of everything I do."

In addition to watching what he eats, Fred runs every day but Sunday, often practicing the distances and events he'll be entering in upcoming track meets.

He says he currently weighs 133 pounds ("I want to get to 130"), and has never had any serious injuries ("Well, aside from a few broken bones and ribs, a lot of pulled hamstrings, and a few teeth knocked out playing football").

But there is much more to Dr. Fred than just wind sprints and 110-meter hurdles. He is, for instance, active on the boards of the Reunion Arena Invitational in Dallas and the Texas Senior Games.

He is also a tireless worker in the fight against muscular dystrophy.

"Our oldest son, my namesake, was born 50 years ago and died of MD at the age of 20," Fred said. "I've been on the muscular dystrophy board for 30 years, and raised an awful lot of money for crippled kids, old folks, wheelchair fellows, everybody. I do it for them."

During the day, Fred can be found on the campus of Dallas Baptist College, where he once served as dean of the division of religion and philosophy.

"Evidently, unless something changes, I'll work as long as I want to at Dallas Baptist," he said. "I officially retired eight years ago when I was 71. When I put the pencil to it, with the annuity from my denomination, Social Security—which I could get at that time—I figured I could have a lot better income by retiring than I could by working full time. And I did want to get rid of the paper shuffling and administrative duties that went with being a dean.

"So I retired officially, but the president said, 'You tell us how much you want to teach, when and what, and tell us what kind of money you want. We'll write up the contract every year accordingly. So that's the way we started out.

"I teach two classes three days a week, I'm still on their insurance program, and I do get a little stipend. It's not much, but I don't need much. Then the fact that I am connected with a university which I dearly love means that I've got the best in all the world. And it doesn't get in the way of running one iota. You just couldn't ask for anything better."

You get the feeling if teaching *does* get in the way of his running, there's going to be a lot of lonely students at Dallas Baptist College some day.

"I run and keep myself in shape, the first thing, because it's right for me," he said. "My physical well-being is a gift. You're not guaranteed, just because you're born, to be born with a good, physically solid body. But I still feel like it is a stewardship obligation *not* to destroy the body you're given.

"Every day I have a good time—every day. I try to see the bright side of every question, and every little irritating thing that happens—I just laugh at it and go on. I don't let it bother me, I don't let it worry me. I just quit all of that. I'm not afraid for my job, I've got a little nest egg laid up. My wife's got a nice big car and she lets me drive it every now and then. I don't worry about it. Life is good—it's not fair a lot of times—but the Lord's good. And He makes the difference."

It quickly becomes obvious to even a casual listener that Fred's strong religious faith is the other driving force in his life.

"When I win a race, I don't try to hide the fact that I'm a Baptist country preacher," he said. "Those people who denigrate that are ignoramuses. I don't try to hide it, but I don't get out and shout it. Those who have known me a long time know where I stand on that sort of thing.

"My whole relation to everything is very deeply spiritual. I just try to live so that I don't violate the principles in which I believe. I don't make any apology about it, but I don't beat anybody else over the head about it, either. I don't try to change the whole world overnight."

The seamless meshing of these twin interests—fitness and faith—has resulted in a man who is at peace with the world, a man who genuinely enjoys life. He laughs long and hard during an interview—generally at his own expense. He is lavish in his praise of his top competitors and not only wishes them well, but wishes there were more of them!

"In a lot of the meets I run against a lot younger runners, generally because we just don't have a lot of runners in their late 70s," he said. "I'd say I have about six or eight fellows I consider serious competitors. So ordinarily, until I get in the regional or national meets, I run against younger men. Now I do prefer to go against men my own age if the competition is worthy. Otherwise, the younger ones can eat your lunch!"

Fred is something of a philosopher. Perhaps it comes from years of lecturing about theology and philosophy. Perhaps it is his wealth of homespun country wisdom. Whatever its source, he is almost always found with a group of people, many of them hanging on to his every word.

One common question asked by young people is, "What can I do to be in great shape when I'm your age, Dr. White?"

"I tell them, 'Take where you are now, get on to do whatever it is you want to do, get all of the advice you can from people who know,'" he said. "Consistency and regularity are the key to it—and stay with it. I wouldn't try to do something you wouldn't enjoy doing because you wouldn't stay with it.

"And I don't believe the saying 'No pain, no gain.' I think that's a fallacy. I've discovered that for myself. I don't train half as hard as I did five years ago, but I have about the same results. I stay in good physical condition without all of that— about as good as I can be at my age.

"So I'd tell young people to get doing something you enjoy doing, be consistent with it, find something you can do by yourself—something that's not conditioned by the weather or whether or not you're with somebody else. Find something you can control yourself, and do it year-round, and stay with it. Get in good condition. And when you get to be my age, there's not any reason on earth—unless something else goes wrong—that you can't go full-blast at it."

Surprisingly, Fred has much the same answer for people in their 50s, 60s—even 70s—who ask a similar question. And the punchline is always the same: "You're never too old to start."

"But the first thing I would I do would be to go to my doctor and get a good physical checkup, heart and everything," he said. "And if I didn't have a doctor who believed in physical exercise, I'd change doctors!

"Then I'd start doing something that I liked to do. I'd start out letting my body talk to me, then I'd gradually work into a full-scale program of physical exercise by doing things I enjoyed that would increase my activity, that would strengthen my body, that would do my heart good. It wouldn't necessarily be running, it might be anything: bicycling, swimming, whatever, so long as there's some activity to it that keeps you moving, and your heart beating. You'll sleep better, eat better, and keep your weight down.

"You're never too old to start, but you need to start where you are. Then you need to get somebody who knows something about it, like your doctor, or somebody else who can give you some pointers so you can maximize what you're trying to do."

Dr. Fred White walks his talk. He maximizes *everything* he does. His no-holds-barred approach spills over into his mental, physical, and spiritual approach to life.

"At meets, I look at these old men my age and say, 'Man, if I can't out-run that scroungy-looking old man, I ought to quit,'" he said. "And they're looking at me and thinking the same thing. The outward appearance is very deceiving. And when the gun goes off, man alive! They're like a cyclone.

"But my mental image is not what I see in the mirror. In my mind when I look in the mirror, I'm about a 9.3 in the 100-meter dash, I'm still a big-chested and flat-stomached senior in college and all of that kind of stuff.

"There's no reason why I can't keep on competing until I get run over by a Mack truck."

It better be a *big* Mack truck.

And the driver *better* keep right on going.

Chapter 25

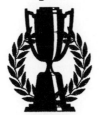

Dexter Woodford

AKRON, OHIO—During the 28.5 miles of the Manhattan Island Marathon, Dexter Woodford was:
* nearly swamped by the wakes from the giant tourist boats of the Circle Line,
* slapped and tossed about by the random waves at the Spuyten Duyvil,
* almost sucked into New York City's mammoth sewer intake channels by the George Washington Bridge,
* on a collision course with a tugboat pushing some giant barges upriver,
* swimming amid various dead animals and "white squishy things,"
* nearly ordered off the race by the Coast Guard, and
* at 77, the oldest man ever to complete one of marathon swimming's most grueling tests.

But Dexter's conquest of the Manhattan Island Marathon pales in comparison to his long-term battle against cancer. His is an incredible story in many ways, the story of a man who seems destined to win *any* contest, no matter what the odds.

Today he is the holder of numerous national records for his age group in a number of freestyle distances. He swims six days a week to get ready for meets. (He sometimes adds a seventh day, just for fun.)

Not surprisingly, Dexter comes from a long line of swimming Woodfords. Older brother Charlie was a pretty fair country swimmer at legendary East High School in Akron, which once won the national long-distance championship in 1935, the only time that title was ever held by something other than a college or men's athletic club.

In 1935, just before entering Ohio State, he won the first

national amateur five-mile swim championship.

At college, Dexter continued his winning ways. He was an All-American in swimming, winning both AAU and NCAA meets during his four years.

"I got married the same year I graduated, then went back to school for two more years to get a master's degree in physics in 1939," Dexter recalled. "Also in 1939, I went through the Work Projects Administration to teach at night. I've always said the degrees after my name should read: B.A., M.A., and WPA.

"In 1940 I got a summer job at Goodyear Research in Akron, where I spent nearly all of the next 40 years—20 of those years in the physics section. During the war, one of my jobs was to finish designing and constructing what would become the first readily available infrared spectrophotometer for examining organic compounds. This led to the development of the better synthetic rubber used during World War II."

Although Dexter did not return to swimming after college, he and his wife Mary became avid sailors, winning numerous regattas on both Lake Erie and Buckeye Lake. In 1944, he was even named commodore of the South Shore Yacht Club.

"When our son Bruce was born in 1952, we at first continued to take him sailing," Dexter said. "But we finally eased out of it because we didn't want to keep worrying about him sliding off the boat! We taught him how to swim pretty early and he ended up especially good in the freestyle and butterfly. At the University of Ohio he held the freshman record for the butterfly for a year or so."

Dexter retired from Goodyear in 1980 at age 64.

"Along about that time, I felt the need for more exercise," he said. "So I started going down to the Y three days a week. It was about then that I discovered the Masters Swimming Program. In short order I was entering the meets, which are divided by age groups. I saw some of the old guys I used to swim against years ago!

"Soon I began practicing more often, usually six days a week, sometimes swimming the two-mile races in Lake Erie. My first competitive YMCA meet came after a year or two of swimming on my own at a YMCA east of Cleveland. I think I won a couple of firsts at that one."

It was as if he had never left. Despite the 40-year layoff, Dexter quickly became the dominant swimmer in his age group.

"I still hold the world records in the 75–79 age group for the 500-, 1,000-, and 1,650-yard dashes," he said. "I also hold the world records in the short course pools in the 400-, 800-, and 1,500-meter distances—all freestyle. I don't currently hold any long course race records, although heaven knows I've tried!"

Along the way, Dexter began to think about swimming the English Channel. The main problem with the Channel is not the distance but the cold water, which defeats even seasoned marathoners. He tried a practice swim at a 2.5-mile race in Indianapolis where the water temperature—60 degrees—approximated that of the English Channel.

"I was all right while I was swimming," he said, "but this was October, mind you, and once I got out in the cold air I got hypothermia—even though they had a tent where they were blowing hot air and they were rubbing the swimmers down. I shivered for 45 minutes—I couldn't stop.

"So I decided against the Channel swim at that time. I would have had to practice a month and a half ahead of time just to get used to it, plus I'd need to get a layer of fat ahead of time. I was still thinking of trying it, but because of my wife's current fragile health, I can't leave her for long periods of time."

His second choice was the Manhattan Island Marathon. Dexter's interest in the Manhattan was piqued when he read an article in 1991 about a swimmer who, at 73, was the oldest man to ever complete the course.

After finishing the article, Dexter thought, "I could do that."

The Manhattan Marathon's course begins at the Battery on the southern tip of Manhattan, goes east, then up the East River to Hell Gate, into the Harlem River, past the Spuyten Dyvil, into the Hudson River, down the Hudson, and finishes back at the Battery. It is 28.5 miles through some of the most polluted, most heavily congested waterways in the world. Dexter could hardly wait.

"I started training in June for the Marathon in nearby Springfield Lake, southeast of Akron," he said. "The first time I swam, I just swam out a little way and swam back to get used to the 73-degree water. The next time I swam across and back. After that, I began swimming one or two miles before motorboats came out. After I got used to that, it wasn't scary at all. Soon I was doing three or four times across the lake and back."

Dexter would begin swimming at 4 or 5 a.m. and try to finish before the water-ski boats roared out at 10 a.m. For most of his swim, he would be in the dark, with only a few ducks or

Canadian geese for company. Within weeks, he was doing up to 11 miles at a stretch.

When the Manhattan Island Marathon began on August 10, 1991, Dexter was one of 41 hardy souls who braved the brackish water.

"My memories of the Marathon were that it wasn't too bad, to begin with, anyway," he said. "I think the worst pollution was in the Harlem River, but the rest wasn't too bad. One of the most interesting things about it was swimming under the Brooklyn Bridge, the Manhattan Bridge, and the Queensboro and Triborough Bridges.

"In the Manhattan Marathon, each swimmer is required to have a manned power boat accompany them with a crew of one or two, to give food and drink, directions, and offer some protection. I also hired a kayaker because there is a railroad bridge near the Spuyten Duyvil where, if there is a train going across, they can't even raise the bridge high enough for a boat to get under. But a kayaker can do it."

"I had a lot of sandwiches I made," he told the *Akron Journal–Beacon*. "I took a whole loaf of Italian deli bread and made honey sandwiches with a fair amount of honey on each one. I cut each one into four pieces so they'd be bite size.

"When I did the 11-mile swim, during the last four miles I got awfully hungry. I didn't get hungry hardly at all in the marathon."

Dexter swam strongly in the early stages of the race, following the kayaker's lead. At one point, the kayaker found a shortcut across the middle of the river, but a Coast Guard patrol boat called out, "You must get closer to the shore!"

"My kayaker said, 'Aw phooey! Don't listen to him, they don't know what they're doing,'" Dexter recalled. "So he kept guiding me along the middle of the river amid all of the big tugboats and barges."

Suddenly, the crew in the power boat got Dexter's attention by using their airhorn.

"My captain said, 'The Coast Guard radioed in if you don't get closer to the shore, he's going to take you out of the water!' And that would be the end of the swim! So I decided to head for the shore, which was about 300–400 yards away. I was all right then—and I eluded one hazard: the Coast Guard!"

Other obstacles were not so easily overcome. In the Harlem River, Dexter saw numerous dead seagulls in the water and a long-dead dog.

"Also about 15–20 times I'd put my hand in the water and pull up these squishy things," Dexter said. "My kayaker said, 'You know what those are? Those are Harlem River White Fish. They grow to about six inches long.' I found out later they were either dead jellyfish—or something else even worse!"

Once past the Hudson River and the Spuyten Duyvil, near the George Washington Bridge, Dexter had to swim against the current of the intake channels for the Manhattan sewage system.

"You can't swim against it; you'd get pulled against some kind of screen there and you can't get away from it," he said. "You'd have to have a boat let a line out to you, tie it around you, and pull you away from it. That's the only way to get away from it. So I was fairly well out in the middle of the river when I went by it, but the intake extends for a quarter of a mile or so! Toward the end I was on my right side passing it. I looked over my left side and I was only 200–300 yards from it. I could see the current going into it."

Dexter managed to pull away from that hazard, but others soon followed. A powerboat apparently didn't see Dexter and only veered away at the last second. A barge on the Hudson nearly blocked the entire waterway. And the huge Circle Line tourist ships, some of which carried as many as 2,000 passengers, threatened to swamp him with their giant wakes each time they passed.

Still, Dexter plunged gamely ahead.

"You just get used to a certain pace," he said. "Just like on our lake out here in Akron, I swim all day to build up some endurance so I can hold on all day. I just keep on going, watching the scenery go by. I tell my friends it is certainly a different way to see New York City! I liked watching the boats going by, the passenger boats with all of the people waving. I liked going by the docks, with the people lining the walkways, watching."

In the end, Dexter was one of 39 swimmers who had completed the marathon. He finished 36th.

"When it was over, I was tired, but I wasn't completely exhausted, even though the last couple of hundred yards I made a dash for the finish," he said. "If I had known that I was that close to nine hours flat, I would have tried even harder! As it was, I finished at nine hours 17 seconds.

"Of course, I haven't entered anything longer than two miles since!"

Unfortunately, the Manhattan Island Marathon apparently

took its toll on Dexter. After the Manhattan, he suffered from diarrhea for six weeks and lost 12 pounds. That was followed by a bout with shingles.

"So a year later I'm still not back; I'm about two-thirds back," he said.

What makes Dexter's swim all the more remarkable is that he is presently in remission from cancer in his left leg. He underwent five major operations and nearly a year's worth of chemotherapy. At one point, doctors tied a tourniquet around the top of the diseased leg. They cut to open an artery, drained the blood, and circulated a concentrated chemical in the limb.

Through it all, Dexter continued to swim.

"I'm sure the swimming has helped to bring back my immune system," he told the *Beacon-Journal.* "It keeps your circulation going."

"My family doctor kind of advised against the long-distance swimming, particularly the marathons. But when I went ahead and did it, he said he was glad. This particular doctor has run in a couple of Boston Marathons, so he understands marathon preparations and requirements. My friends have been encouraging, too."

Dexter's friends come in various ages.

"I like swimming with people of all ages," he said. "I like making a lot of friends and you never saw a healthier, happier bunch of people than swimmers.

"I'm also in a group called Research Retirees and we meet once a month. We recently had a meeting at a restaurant about seven miles away. On my 75th birthday, I walked three miles down to the water, swam four miles, and met them at the restaurant!"

Whether dining in restaurants or at home, Dexter says he is conscious of what he eats.

"I eat a pretty good breakfast," he said. "My wife watches our diet pretty well and I owe a lot to her for keeping us in good health. Three days a week we eat boiled oats, always orange juice, bananas, buttered toast and jelly, and I take an aspirin a day. We used to drink a couple cups of coffee. For a while I cut that out altogether, but now I'm back to one cup a day.

"After that big breakfast, for lunch we'll have soup or a sandwich and maybe some fruit.

"And for supper, maybe a salad, maybe some various things. We're not vegetarians, although we eat a lot more vegetables than meat. And we usually eat chicken or fish.

In his spare time, Dexter set up The Woodford Tool & Instrument Co. in his basement, and crafts a small number of handmade tools and instruments for other small industries.

"My primary hobby is my machine shop, and it is something that grew into a paying hobby," he said. "I turned in a $250 job last week and I'm working a six-piece job at $300 each that I have to get done this month."

But mostly, Dexter swims. His accomplishments have been written up in *Sports Illustrated* and *USA Today*, but he modestly downplays them.

"I try to be an inspiration to other people," he said. "In my daily life, I just try to do what I have to do each day."

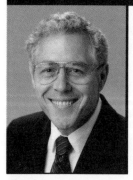

This book was born when I was watching a commercial on TV and saw 83-year-old Banana George barefoot skiing. I told my wife to come and see this "December champion." I liked the name so much I recruited Bob Darden to go to work on this book, as an inspiration for the fastest-growing group of Americans—active seniors. I'm 58 myself, and my secret ambition is to be a character in an updated version of December Champions *when I'm about 75.*

W. R. Spence, M.D.
Publisher

*T*he book division of WRS Publishing focuses on true stories about everyday heroes, like these December champions, who have accomplished their own impossible dreams. While it is often easy to turn a profit with stories of greed, sex, and violence, we are not interested in such books. We only produce books we can be proud of and that can change lives for the better. **Call us at 1-800-299-3366 for suggestions or for a free book catalog.**

WATCH FOR THESE RELATED TITLES:

TEN MILLION STEPS is the story of Paul Reese, who ran across America—a marathon a day for 170 days—at age 73.

YOUNG AT HEART outlines the running career of 85-year-old Johnny Kelley—who has answered the starting gun at 63 Boston Marathons—and of long-distance running in America in this century.

THE MAN WHO WOULD NOT BE DEFEATED tells of W Mitchell, who has triumphed over two life-threatening accidents that left him scarred and paralyzed.

NO LIMITS is the inspiring story of Harry Cordellos, blind runner, skier, triathlete, and role model.

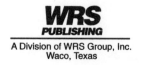

WRS
PUBLISHING

A Division of WRS Group, Inc.
Waco, Texas